D1824232

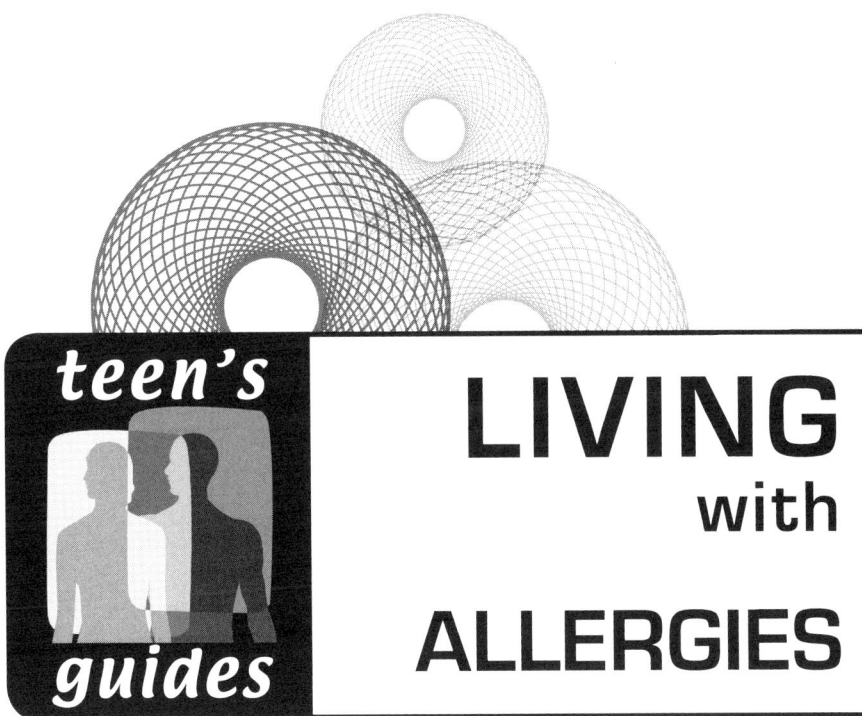

teen's guides

guides

LIVING
with
ALLERGIES

Also in the
Teen's Guides series

teen's guides

LIVING
with
ALLERGIES

Paul M. Ehrlich, M.D.
with
Elizabeth Shimer Bowers

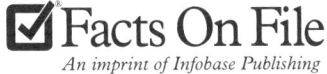

✓Facts On File
An imprint of Infobase Publishing

Living with Allergies

Copyright © 2009 by Paul M. Ehrlich, M.D.

Facts On File, Inc.
An imprint of Infobase Publishing, Inc.
132 West 31st Street
New York NY 10001

Library of Congress Cataloging-in-Publication Data

Ehrlich, Paul M.
    Living with allergies / by Paul M. Ehrich, with Elizabeth Shimer.
      p. cm — (Living with allergies)
    Includes bibliographical references and index.
    ISBN-13: 978-0-8160-7327-6 (alk. paper)
    ISBN-10: 0-8160-7327-9 (alk. paper)
  1. Allergy. I. Bowers, Elizabeth Shimer. II. Title.
    RC584.E37   2007
    616.97—dc22   2008034352

Facts On File books are available at special discounts when purchased in bulk quantities for businesses, associations, institutions, or sales promotions. Please call our Special Sales Department in New York at (212) 967-8800 or (800) 322-8755.

You can find Facts On File on the World Wide Web at http://www.factsonfile.com

Text design by Annie O'Donnell
Cover design by Jooyoung An

Printed in the United States of America

Sheridan Hermitage 10 9 8 7 6 5 4 3 2 1

This book is printed on acid-free paper.

CONTENTS

What Are Allergies?

To Paul, 15, peanuts are like poison. When his mom fed him peanut butter for the first time when he was five, his throat closed, and he nearly died. At the hospital, doctors gave Paul an *adrenaline* shot and told his mother that he had a severe *peanut allergy* and would have to avoid contact with peanuts and nuts for the rest of his life. Even a tiny speck of food containing peanuts could be deadly to him.

Since then, Paul has accidentally encountered peanuts on a few different occasions, and he was sent to the emergency room each time. When he is exposed to a nut, Paul immediately feels a tight, tingling sensation in his mouth and throat. He then develops *hives* on his skin, and his lips become hot and swollen. In sensitive people like Paul, peanut and nut allergies can trigger swelling of the mouth and throat, low blood pressure, spasms in their breathing tubes, and *anaphylactic shock.*

The last time Paul had a reaction, he was in the cafeteria at school. Someone at his lunch table opened a bag of peanuts, and the dust from the nuts triggered an attack. Paul swelled up immediately, and an ambulance came for him. Once he arrived at the hospital, a shot of adrenaline saved Paul once again.

Paul has been lucky: Each time he has been exposed to peanuts and suffered a reaction, he has gotten to the hospital in time, but other teenagers with similar allergies have not been so fortunate. Recent news stories have made the public more aware of how sensitive some patients with peanut and nut allergies really are. According to the Food Allergy and Anaphylaxis Network, teens with peanut and nut allergies are at the highest risk for a fatal reaction for a few reasons: They might not recognize early symptoms; they may not have the appropriate medication with them; and their friends may not realize the severity of the situation and therefore not call for help fast enough. They may also have *asthma,* which can exacerbate the problem.

The good news is that there are some things Paul—and you, if you have allergies—can do to ease his mind and the worried minds of his parents and friends. For one, Paul can carry a *Twinject* or *EpiPen.* These are prescription-strength *epinephrine* auto-injectors that teenagers with severe allergies can carry with them in case they suffer an emergency attack. Paul knows what foods he can safely eat and which ones to avoid. He also makes sure to inform new friends about the issue. Because he is armed with knowledge about how to safely manage his allergy, Paul leads a pretty normal life as a teenager.

Of course, relatively few people have a life-threatening reaction like Paul's. It's much more likely that you or your friends have a more common allergic reaction, like sneezing fits or a stuffy nose during "*pollen* season" in early spring. Both kinds of reactions—and many more—are symptoms of what doctors call *allergies.*

WHAT IS AN ALLERGY?

The word *allergy* comes from the Greek word *allos,* which means "an altered state." An allergy is your *immune system*'s abnormal response to things that are harmless to other people. When you are allergic to something, your immune system thinks the substance—food, *dust,* pollen, medicines, and so on—is harmful to your body. In response, it sends off a false alarm in the form of an allergic reaction.

More specifically, in an attempt to protect your body from the substance it thinks is harmful, your immune system produces what are known as *IgE antibodies* to that *allergen.* These *antibodies* cause certain cells in your body to release chemicals into your bloodstream, including *cytokines, leukotrienes,* and a chemical called *histamine.* This histamine is what causes the annoying reaction in your eyes, nose, throat, lungs, skin, or intestinal tract, which is why you take a medication called an *antihistamine* to make the allergic reaction stop.

It works like this: When you are approached by a bacteria or something foreign, you produce an antibody against it. Then the next time your body encounters that substance, the antibodies attack it before it can produce any symptoms. In nonallergic people, DNA is not programmed to produce the IgE antibody. These people can smother themselves with peanut butter and not have a problem. If, however, you are programmed to produce IgE antibodies in response to that particular substance, you will have a reaction. The IgE antibodies have claws like lobsters. The dust, *mold,* or other allergen fits into those claws and forms a bridge that allows the allergens into your bloodstream where they can wreak havoc.

An important part of the allergic reaction is a cell called a *mast cell.* Mast cells are like a combined command center and military base for your body. When you encounter a substance you are allergic to, the IgE antibodies hook on to mast cells—about 10,000 IgE molecules per mast cell—and the mast cells take on water, swell, and burst, releasing the histamine that causes hives, itching, sneezing, and other annoying allergy symptoms. You have mast cells all over your body—in your skin, *respiratory system,* eyes, and gastrointestinal tract—which is why allergic reactions can occur in all these areas.

You can think of an allergic reaction in your immune system like a guard dog; your immune system means well, but it becomes confused and reacts inappropriately. When it is properly trained and in its proper place, a guard dog offers protection against invaders (or, in the case of the immune system, bacteria and viruses). However, allergies are like guard dogs turned loose in a residential neighborhood—any innocent thing that comes across their path is in great danger.

What's more, your immune system has a memory. Each time your immune system comes across an allergen, it produces more antibodies faster than the time before. Different chain reactions occur in response to the dust, mold, pollen, food, or other thing to which you are allergic. Some of these chain reactions are merely annoying, and others are very dangerous.

Milder allergic reactions come in the form of slightly itchy eyes, a runny nose, itchy throat, or other uncomfortable symptoms. Severe allergic reactions, on the other hand, can threaten your life and should be taken seriously. The most severe allergic reaction is called *anaphylaxis,* which involves difficulty breathing, difficulty swallowing, dizziness or passing out, and swelling of the lips, tongue, throat, or other parts of the body. Anaphylaxis, which is the reaction Paul and others with peanut allergies experience after eating nuts, usually happens minutes after you've been exposed to an allergen, but it can also be delayed for as long as four hours. Luckily, these severe anaphylactic allergic reactions are rare, and they can be successfully treated if you follow the proper medical procedures.

Overall, allergies are fairly common, and they occur equally in males and females. They affect as many as 60 million Americans, or one in five people. The most common allergen is airborne pollen, which gives 35 million people upper respiratory symptoms. The second most common allergen is cats, with 10 million sufferers, followed by insect stings, which cause allergies in 2 million Americans. Food allergies are less common; although one in three people *think* they have a food allergy, only about 3 to 8 percent of children under three years old and 1 percent of adults actually have allergies to foods.

THE HISTORY OF ALLERGIES

As long as there have been human beings, it appears that there have been human beings with allergies. Roman philosopher Lucretius was one of the first to describe allergies, saying, "what is good for some may be fierce poisons for others." For King Menses of Egypt, a wasp sting was most definitely poison—the king died after being stung by a wasp some time between 3640 and 3300 B.C. Another allergy sufferer was the Roman Emperor Claudius's son Britannicus, who developed a rash and swollen eyes after being around horses. Legend has it that King Richard III used his own allergy to strawberries to murder his enemy, Lord William Hastings. The king purposely ate some strawberries just prior to being around Hastings and then blamed his allergic reaction on a curse from the lord; as a result, Lord Hastings was beheaded.

As far as the medical community is concerned, *hay fever*—an allergy affecting more than 15 million Americans that causes sneezing, a runny and stuffed nose, and itchy eyes and throat—was the first allergy to be recognized. In 1819, Dr. John Bostock described hay fever as a disease of the respiratory tract. Then, in 1869, Dr. Charles Blakely performed the first allergy *skin test* by putting pollen into a small cut on his skin. Blakely found that a rash that developed about 20 minutes after the test meant he was indeed allergic to the pollen.

In 1902, vaccine researchers Charles Richet and Paul Portier invented the word anaphylaxis to describe the serious allergic reaction. Shortly after, in 1906, Austrian pediatrician Clemens von Pirquet used the word allergy for the first time to describe the reaction some of his patients had to a certain medicine. *Allergy shots* first made their debut in 1937 thanks to scientists Leonard Noon and John Freeman, and Daniel Bovet created the first antihistamine drug after he and his fellow scientists found that they could block the histamine that created the sneezing, hives, and other allergy symptoms.

Since then, additional advancements in the area of allergy research have taken place, including the development of allergy drugs called *corticosteroids,* discovery of the mast cell, and detection of the role of IgE antibodies. In the early 1980s, Professor Bengt I. Samuelsson received the Nobel Prize in Medicine/Physiology after he identified substances called leukotrienes as the main cause of anaphylaxis. His finding expanded scientists' knowledge of allergy significantly.

THE CAUSES OF ALLERGIES

Although people have been suffering from allergies for thousands of years, scientists have only recently begun to understand *why* they occur. One theory suggests that allergies might be a leftover survival tactic. In the days when people lived on the banks of the Tigris and Euphrates Rivers, they came across many parasites, and their immune systems needed to be powerful to fight off the invaders they came across on a daily basis. Some people's immune systems responded better than others to the parasites and produced more IgE, and these people survived. So, long ago, being an allergic person may have been an advantage.

Today, however, few people live on the banks of a river where parasites are a threat. In fact, most of us wear shoes that keep parasites from entering through our feet, live in sealed air-conditioned buildings, sleep under synthetic covers, and eat fruits and vegetables treated with pesticides. Thanks to climate control, modern sanitation, and vaccines, we don't face the same problems as our ancestors. However, our bodies are still ready for action, and because our immune systems' natural tendency to fight invaders have nothing to really combat, they react to things that are actually not a threat—dust on the windowsill, mold in the basement, Fluffy the cat. Plus, our wall-to-wall carpeting and throw rugs create areas where dust and *dust mites* thrive. In a way, allergies are the price we pay for progress, and we are suffering from allergies at higher numbers than ever before.

Modern conveniences aside, it seems that allergies are one case where it may be okay to point the finger at Mom or Dad, because in many cases, allergies are passed down from them. However, just because your mom, dad, sister, or brother suffers from allergies doesn't necessarily mean you're doomed to get them too. If one of your parents has allergies, the odds are in your favor; you have only about a 20 to 30 percent chance of developing them yourself. If both of your parents have allergies, the chances are more like 70 percent.

Although the tendency to have allergies may come from your parents, specific allergies usually do not. Your dad may be allergic to cats and mold, while you may sneeze after exposure to dogs and pollen. You may not develop an allergy until you reach your later teens or adult years, after your system has been repeatedly exposed to an allergen and therefore sensitized to it. The more you are exposed to a potential allergen—for example, pollen—the more antibodies build up until one day they are released in an allergic reaction.

For many years, researchers thought allergies were only short-term events. After being around pollen, mold, or a cat, a person would get itchy eyes and a runny nose, and then the reaction would go away in a few hours. Scientists also thought that the only reason for these symptoms was the toxin histamine, which is why antihistamine medications have traditionally been the first medication used to treat allergies.

Today, scientists realize that allergies may not be so simple. It seems that histamine not only rises to fight the allergen but also causes a chain reaction of other events. In addition to histamine, mast cells produce leukotrienes and substances known as cytokines, which stimulate inflammation and damage healthy tissue. Allergies may do more than just cause annoying sneezing and runny nose symptoms for a few hours; they may also lead to medical problems years down the road. It seems that over time, if you do not treat your allergies, they may permanently damage cells in your body, which is why it's so important for you to keep your allergies under control.

SYMPTOMS OF ALLERGIES

The symptoms of allergies vary widely—some are merely bothersome and others are life threatening. For example, one person may get a few hives after eating a food he is allergic to, while another may stop breathing. With that being said, allergy symptoms tend to follow somewhat of a pattern, with certain allergens producing distinctive reactions. The most common reactions to allergens are congestion, *wheezing,* sneezing, itchy eyes, skin irritation or itchiness, and hives. More specifically, if you have allergies, you may experience one or more of the following symptoms:

Food and drug allergy symptoms
- Wheezing (a whistling or hissing sound when breathing out, caused by narrowed airways), shortness of breath, chest tightness
- Itchy mouth
- Trouble swallowing

➤ Diarrhea or vomiting

➤ Abdominal pain

➤ Hives (red, itchy, swollen areas on the skin), skin itching, or rash

Airborne allergen symptoms (such as dust and pollen)

➤ Runny or stuffy nose

➤ Sneezing

➤ Coughing

➤ Itchy eyes, nose, and throat

➤ Watery eyes

➤ Dark circles under the eyes (caused by increased blood flow near your sinuses)

➤ Wheezing, chest tightness, shortness of breath

➤ *Conjunctivitis,* or inflammation of the membranes that line your eyelids

HOW ALLERGIES AFFECT DAILY LIFE

If you suffer from allergies, you know better than anyone how they affect you. You are probably sick more often than your friends, which may make you feel angry or frustrated at times. If you have a food allergy, you probably have to constantly watch the foods you eat and read ingredient labels, which can grow tiresome. Sometimes you may also feel guilty because your allergies interfere with the activities you do with your friends and family. You occasionally may feel anxious or depressed because of the toll your allergies take on your day-to-day activities. All these emotions are very common in teens who suffer from allergies, so you are certainly not alone.

You may also notice that your allergies have interfered more and more with your daily life as you've gotten into your teenage years. As a teen, you are probably becoming more involved with activities in and out of school, and your allergies may get in the way sometimes. In elementary school, you knew all your classmates well, and they were aware of your allergy. In middle school and high school, things change a little. You are introduced to new classmates and teachers to whom you have to explain your allergy.

In addition, as you are getting older, you have greater freedom from your parents. You probably spend more time with your friends, eat more junk food, and you may have started dating. These are rights of passage as a teenager, but they also expose you to new people and environments and, therefore, more opportunities to encounter the things you are allergic to. As you approach adulthood, you have more responsibility to avoid allergens and to educate people around you about what to do if you have an attack. If you feel confused or ill-equipped to handle the new freedom that goes along with being a teenager, talk to your parents, your family physician, or your *allergist*. They will give you the knowledge and advice you need to feel more comfortable in new situations, and they will give you the tools necessary to deal with an attack should one take place.

SOCIAL REPERCUSSIONS OF ALLERGIES

In your teenage years, you face new social situations. As a teen with allergies, you face special challenges, which can lead to some stress and anxiety now and then. You have more peers in school than ever before, and your friends and classmates may form exclusive groups or cliques. As a result, the pressure to fit in is enormous. At this time in your life, your allergies may feel like more of a burden than they did in the past, and you may feel as though you are different from other kids your age. Your sneezing or sniffling may become distracting, and your friends and classmates may tease you about it. If you have a food allergy, you may have to sit away from your classmates until they understand what they can and cannot open and eat near you.

Your allergies may also interfere with social activities you engage in outside of school, such as hanging out with friends at a mall or coffee shop, or attending a birthday party or bar mitzvah. For example, if you and your friends go out for ice cream and you are allergic to nuts, you will have to request that others skip the peanuts on their sundaes. At parties, you may have to refrain from eating some of the food to avoid accidental exposure to an allergen. These situations may cause you to feel lonely and out of place at times, which is a perfectly normal and understandable reaction.

Because you will be hanging out with your friends more often, it's your responsibility as a teenager with allergies to inform them about your allergy and how they can help you avoid accidental exposure and deal with an emergency should one occur. If you have a food allergy, for example, tell each and every one of your friends. If you are dating, before you engage in kissing, talk to your partner about your food allergy—even if you didn't eat the food yourself, a residual amount of it in your partner's mouth can trigger a reaction in you. If you are sexually active and have a *latex* allergy, tell your partner about your need to use a nonlatex condom. True friends and loyal boyfriends/girlfriends will be sympathetic and understanding about your situation, and they will do whatever they can to protect you.

Another issue surrounding allergies that can interfere with your social life as a teenager is carrying your medications. If you're a girl, you can easily carry your meds in a purse, but if you are a boy, it may be a little more challenging. In middle and high school, you are probably concerned about looking "nerdy," and a pocket full of medication certainly doesn't help the situation. One good solution may be to wear cargo pants or shorts with lots of pockets to hold medication or injectors. Or, you can carry a backpack, attaché case, or messenger bag with you at all times, and stick your medications in the bag.

Of course your allergies come into play when you are preparing to leave for a family vacation or summer camp. To best prepare for all possible situations, you will have to carefully pack all your medications and supplies, and you and your parents will need to make sure all traveling companions and camp counselors know about your allergy and what to do in the event of an attack. As a teenager with allergies, there is no reason you can't do all the things your nonallergic friends do—you just need to take some extra precautions.

HOW FRIENDS SHOULD DEAL WITH ALLERGIES

If you have a friend with allergies, there are a few things you can do to make him or her feel as normal, safe, and comfortable as possible. It is a delicate balance—you don't want to make your friend feel different, but at the same time, if you are not aware of what can happen during an allergy attack, or if you are not prepared to handle an attack should one occur, the consequences can be dire. That's why it is crucial that you know the details of your friend's allergy so you can recognize when a reaction occurs and respond appropriately in an allergic emergency.

For one, if your friend is carrying an auto-injector device such as a Twinject or EpiPen, make sure you know how to use it and where he or she is carrying it at all times. That way, should an allergy attack take place, you can get to the device quickly and administer a dose. There is a device available called an EpiPen Trainer—it contains no needle or drug, and it is a great training tool for how to use an EpiPen in the event of a real allergy emergency.

Next, if your friend has a food allergy, don't be afraid to ask questions; inquire about which foods he or she is allergic to, what will happen if he or she is exposed to those foods, and what you should do to help in the event of an attack. If you notice that your friend is becoming lax about reading ingredients labels or asking cafeteria employees about ingredients in prepared foods, gently remind him about the seriousness of his condition. Or, if he leaves his EpiPen in his locker at lunch and resists going back to get it, encourage him to do so or offer to go get it for him. After all, friends are some of the strongest influencers on each others' lives in the teenage years. Your friend may respond negatively at first, but he will be thankful in the long run.

CONDUCTING AN ALLERGY SELF-EVALUATION

If you suspect you may have an allergy but you're not sure, here is an allergy self-evaluation from the Allergy Institute to help you find out. Answer the following questions to find out if you have an allergy or another condition:

1. I have a stuffy nose, runny nose, postnasal drip, or nasal itching at least one month of each year. Yes or No
2. I have itchy, dry, irritated, or watery eyes and swollen eyelids sometimes. Yes or No
3. My nose or ears feel plugged often even though I don't have a cold. Yes or No
4. I sometimes have yellow or green mucous. Yes or No
5. I often feel like my nose is blocked at night, and I have started snoring. Yes or No
6. I have missed school because of allergies, sinus problems, or trouble with breathing. Yes or No
7. I have had surgery to correct a sinus problem, deviated septum, or for ear tubes. Yes or No
8. I have taken antibiotics numerous times for chest, ear, or sinus infections in the past year. Yes or No
9. I avoid some activities I used to enjoy because of allergy symptoms. Yes or No

If you answered *Yes* to more than five of these questions, you may suffer from allergies. Talk to your family doctor about your symptoms or make an appointment with an allergy specialist who can evaluate the problem and develop an effective treatment plan.

WHAT YOU NEED TO KNOW

If you have allergies or have a friend or family member with allergies, here are some facts you should know:

▶ Allergies are the third leading cause of chronic disease in the country, ahead of diabetes, cancer, coronary heart disease, and stroke.

Allergy Warning Signs

As an allergy sufferer, you probably know the symptoms that indicate a pending attack, but there are certain warning signs that may signal a more serious type of allergic reaction—signs you should be aware of so you are ready to fight back in case they strike.

The most serious allergic reaction is anaphylaxis, which is marked by hives, swelling, lowered blood pressure, and dilated blood vessels. The allergens that most frequently cause anaphylaxis are foods such as shellfish (lobster, shrimp), nuts, sesame seeds, egg whites, dairy products, and bee stings. Other substances can cause a similar reaction to anaphylaxis called an *anaphylactoid reaction,* which is just as serious as anaphylaxis but does not involve IgE. Allergens that can cause anaphylactoid reactions include fish, latex, and some medications, like penicillin. If anaphylaxis is not treated immediately, the person suffering from it can go into shock and possibly even die.

The initial warning signs of anaphylaxis include:

▶ Difficulty breathing

▶ Wheezing (a whistling or hissing sound when breathing out, caused by narrowed airways)

▶ Difficulty swallowing

▶ Confusion

▶ Slurred speech

▶ Rapid or weak pulse

▶ Blueness of the skin, including the lips or nail beds

▶ Fainting, lightheadedness, or dizziness

▶ Anxiety

▶ Heart palpitations (feeling your heart beating)

▶ Severe itching of the eyes and face

▶ Hives

(continues)

(continued)

> Abdominal pain and cramping

> Vomiting and/or diarrhea

> Nasal congestion

> Coughing

If you experience any of these symptoms of anaphylaxis, it is important that you seek medical attention right away. If you are allergic to bee stings, nuts, or other substances that can cause anaphylaxis, you should always be prepared for an attack. Carry an epinephrine injection kit such as a Twinject or EpiPen at all times, and for maximum protection, wear a MedicAlert bracelet or pendant or carry a card that alerts others of your allergy in the case of an emergency. When it comes to your allergy, you cannot take too many precautions. Planning ahead could make the difference between life and death.

> Seventy-five percent of allergy sufferers have what are termed indoor/outdoor allergies, which produce allergic *rhinitis,* hay fever, and nasal allergies.
> Allergies account for 17 million outpatient physician visits per year, half of which are due to seasonal allergies.
> Skin allergies account for more than 7 million outpatients per year.
> The most common allergens are pollen, mold spores, animal *dander,* dust mite and cockroach allergen, and insect stings.
> If you are allergic to pollen, you will have trouble avoiding it—the pollens of some grasses, trees, and plants are so light that they can travel for up to 400 miles out at sea and two miles into the atmosphere.
> About 7 percent of allergy sufferers have skin allergies as their primary allergy, and the most common skin allergy triggers are plants such as poison ivy, poison oak, and poison sumac.

However, certain foods, latex, and cockroach and dust mite allergen may also cause skin reactions.

➤ An estimated 6 percent of allergy sufferers are allergic to foods or drugs. Food allergies can be very serious, causing about 200 deaths per year in this country.

➤ Approximately 4 percent of allergy sufferers have latex as their primary allergy, and 10 percent of health-care workers are allergic to latex.

➤ About 4 percent of allergy sufferers have insect bites as their primary allergy (allergies to bee, wasp, and venomous ant bites; dust mite and cockroach allergen can also cause nasal or skin reactions).

➤ Approximately 4 percent of allergy sufferers have eye allergies (also called allergic conjunctivitis or ocular allergies) as their primary allergies. Eye allergies are usually caused by many of the same triggers as indoor/outdoor allergies.

➤ If you have an allergy as a teenager, you may outgrow it for a while or permanently. In teenage boys with allergies, 30 to 50 percent lose their allergies, but some return once they have reached 40. Girls, on the other hand, often do not develop allergies until their late teens.

➤ Although pets and dust mites are commonly identified as allergens, there are some myths surrounding them. It's actually the waste matter of dust mites—not the mites themselves—that cause the allergic reaction. And in the case of furry animals, it's not their fur but the proteins secreted by skin glands that are found in the dander, the proteins in the saliva that stick to the animal's fur when it licks itself, and the proteins found in their urine that make you sneeze and sniffle.

➤ No matter what your allergy, you are not doomed to an existence filled with dust masks, restricted diet, or a pet-free household. With the right information from your health care professionals and resources like this book, you can live a relatively normal life. The secret is to educate yourself and always be prepared.

2

Is It Really an Allergy? Getting a Diagnosis

Now that you have a clearer understanding of what an allergy is, you might be wondering whether your irritating itchy eyes or relentless runny nose are the result of an allergy and not just your run-of-the-mill springtime cold. Although allergies are more prevalent in society than ever, the phrase, "I am allergic to . . ." is thrown around far too loosely. Many teens—and adults, for that matter—will point the finger at allergies for the reactions they get in response to things like cigarette smoke, paint fumes, plastics, temperature changes, perfumes, and more. Although these things in the environment do cause an annoying reaction, they do not cause allergy symptoms in the true sense of the word. Similarly, food intolerances, such as the inability to digest wheat gluten or milk, or sensitivity to the food preservative monosodium glutamate (MSG), are not true food allergies, but they are often falsely blamed as such.

Furthermore, even when patients have correctly diagnosed themselves with an allergy, they are often wrong about what it is that they are allergic to. They might point the finger at pollen, when Fido or Gigi the cat may actually be to blame. This chapter will help you better understand whether or not you have an allergy, guide you in the right direction for a concrete diagnosis, and offer some tools to help you better deal with your allergy should you be diagnosed with one.

IS IT ALLERGIES?

Ironically, the more serious allergies, such as Paul's allergy to peanuts, are often the easiest to diagnose. An anaphylactic reaction is always the result of an allergy. Other allergy symptoms, like the ones that accompany hay fever, are a little harder to decipher.

Perhaps the most frequently confused ailments are allergies and colds. Since both allergies and colds produce sneezing, itchy and watery eyes, and a runny nose, it can be hard to pinpoint the true nature of the problem. However, if you know what to look for, there are some fairly easy ways to distinguish the two. First, in addition to the sniffling and sneezing, colds may also produce colored mucus, a fever, and aches and pains. Allergies strike in the spring, summer, and fall and linger for weeks to months, while colds occur more often in the winter (although they can strike at any time), and they usually only last a week or so.

Although it may seem harmless to call a cold or food intolerance an allergy, it is actually pretty important that you get a correct allergy diagnosis so you can receive proper treatment. Allergies often strike people for the first time in the teenage years, so as a teen, if you experience any new sniffles, sneezes, or hives, you should be checked. And you should seek treatment for any cold symptoms that last more than two weeks because these symptoms can lead to sinusitis, a condition that needs to be treated more aggressively.

In addition, here are some other symptoms that indicate you should probably pay a visit to the doctor:

- ▸ You have frequent allergy attacks that interfere with school or work.
- ▸ You experience sniffling and sneezing that interfere with your life and/or lead to sinus infections often.
- ▸ You have had a severe reaction to a bee sting, mosquito bite, or other insect bite.
- ▸ You have been hospitalized for an asthma attack.
- ▸ Medications (either prescribed or *over-the-counter*) are not helpful in treating your allergy symptoms, or they produce unpleasant side effects.
- ▸ You get frequent skin rashes, especially rashes that itch.
- ▸ You experience hives or swelling.
- ▸ You have any food allergy symptoms, mild or severe.
- ▸ You are tired of your symptoms and looking for a solution, even if that means allergy shots.

WHERE TO GO FOR ALLERGY DIAGNOSIS

If you or your parents suspect you might have an allergy, your first step should be to decide where to go for a diagnosis. Sit down with your parents or guardian to discuss where you should go, be it your family doctor or a doctor who specializes in treating allergies, called an allergist. You may decide to make an appointment with your family doctor first, and this can be a good way to go. Some insurance companies require that you go to a family doctor as a first step anyway, and your family doctor may be able to rule out allergies based on your symptoms alone.

If your family physician suspects you might have an allergy, he or she may do a few allergy tests (some family physicians do allergy testing in their offices) or refer you to an allergist or to another specialist such as a *dermatologist, otolaryngologist* (ear, nose, and throat doctor), *pulmonologist* (lung specialist), or *rheumatologist.*

In addition to those mentioned above, you should also consider the following factors when you and your parents make the decision to go to your family physician or an allergist. Most general practitioners can conduct allergy tests and review the results, but they may not be as knowledgeable as allergists about when those tests should be ordered and when they should not. Allergy tests are important, but they are not always required. Plus, a good allergist will know which questions to ask, which questions to skip, and how to interpret the symptoms that you and your parents describe. They are familiar with the complex range of things in your environment and your genes that can cause allergies. Allergists receive training in internal medicine and they then go through additional training in the immune system and learn special techniques in treating allergies.

On the other hand, it is more expensive to go directly to an allergist, and unless you want to pay out of pocket, it may not be possible if your insurance company requires a referral from your family doctor. You should discuss all these issues with your parents in order to make the best decision about whether to see your family physician or an allergist for your symptoms.

WHAT TO LOOK FOR IN AN ALLERGY SPECIALIST

If you and your parents decide to go the route of an allergist to diagnose your allergies, you want to make sure you find the best possible man or woman for the job. To find a qualified allergist in your area, you can start by asking your family physician whom he or she recommends. Even if you don't go through your family doctor for a referral, he may know an allergist he trusts and respects.

Beyond your family physician, you can start by looking in the phone book under "physicians." Physicians will be listed under specialties, such as "allergy and immunology." You can also write or call either the American Academy of Allergy, Asthma & Immunology or the American College of Allergy, Asthma & Immunology by using the contact information in the appendix at the back of this book. Both the American Academy of Allergy, Asthma & Immunology (AAAAI) and the American College of Allergy, Asthma & Immunology (ACAAI) are professional organizations representing allergists in the United States.

No matter how you find an allergist, make sure he or she is board certified. In order to become board certified, an allergist must pass a challenging exam, proving that he is competent in the field of allergies. Board-certified allergists have certifications from the American Board of Internal Medicine (ABIM) and/or the American Board of Pediatrics (ABP), followed by additional certification by the American Board of Allergy and Immunology (ABAI). Some allergists have more than one board certification, meaning they have passed tests from multiple boards. Board-certified allergists have the most complete knowledge of the causes and treatments for allergies, so you will receive the best care from them.

BEFORE YOU GO TO THE DOCTOR

You can make things go more smoothly at your doctor's visit by doing some preparation beforehand. Think about your allergy symptoms and how they have interfered with your life recently. Write down all the symptoms you can recall and the instances when they have plagued you. To help you remember all the points you should bring up at your appointment, here is a guide based on questions the doctor is likely to ask:

- What are your symptoms?
- How long ago did your symptoms begin?
- What do you think is causing your symptoms?
- Do your symptoms occur year-round or just in certain months?
- Does eating certain types of foods or being around pets cause your allergy symptoms to flare?
- How long do your symptoms last?
- What makes your symptoms get worse? What makes them get better?

➤ Do allergies run in your family?
➤ What allergies have you been tested for in the past, if any?
➤ Have you ever been hospitalized for an allergic reaction or symptoms you thought may have been the result of an allergy?
➤ Are you taking any prescription or over-the-counter drugs to treat your symptoms? If so, what are they? Have they helped?
➤ Are you taking any herbal supplements? If so, what are they? Have they helped?
➤ Are you allergic to any drugs?

In addition, prepare a list of questions that you want to ask the doctor. Here are some suggestions as to questions you might want to ask:

➤ What might I be allergic to?
➤ What kinds of tests are you going to perform to diagnose my allergy?
➤ Where can I go to learn more about my allergy?
➤ What areas of my body will be affected by my allergy and how?
➤ How might my allergy get in the way of my everyday activities?
➤ What is the long-term outlook for my allergy?
➤ What are my treatment options? Will I be treated regularly or on an as-needed basis?
➤ What can I do on my own to help the problem?
➤ How will special circumstances in my life be affected by my allergies? (These circumstances may include exercise, school life, sports, home environment, eating in the cafeteria, eating out, pets, pregnancy, surgery, and so on.)
➤ Regarding my medications, how much should I take and for how long? How will I know if the medications are working?
➤ What are the side effects of the medication? How might it interfere with other medications I am taking?
➤ What should I do if I forget to take my medication?
➤ How do I know when I can treat my symptoms on my own? How will I be able to tell whether I should just make an office appointment versus going to the emergency room? What can I do if symptoms strike on a weekend or in the middle of the night?
➤ If you have asthma, ask your doctor to give you an asthma care plan.

Ten Questions To Ask
Your Allergy Professional

These days, most physicians don't have much time to spend with each individual patient. So the more prepared you are with questions before your visit, the better. For the sake of time, here are the 10 most important questions for you to ask your physician:

1) Based on my symptoms, what do you think I am allergic to?

2) What kinds of tests can I expect?

3) How might my allergy get in the way of my everyday activities?

4) What are my treatment options?

5) What can I do on my own to help the problem?

6) When should I go to the emergency room?

7) Where can I go to learn more about allergies?

8) What kind of medications might you prescribe?

9) What are the side effects?

10) Which over-the-counter medications can I take to ease my symptoms?

In addition, you can better prepare for your doctor's visit by putting together a symptom diary. When you experience symptoms, record when they occurred, what you were doing when they took place, what the weather was like, any odors or smells you noticed, and what you suspected caused the attack. The longer you can record symptoms in your symptom diary before you have your appointment, the better. You should not, however, put off an appointment in order to log more symptoms in your diary. If you are having allergy symptoms, you should get to the doctor for a diagnosis as soon as possible.

ALLERGY TESTS

The health care professional you will see for your allergies is no doubt extremely knowledgeable, but he or she does not have a magic crystal ball. Therefore, he may need to administer some allergy tests before giving you a definitive diagnosis. Allergy testing is particularly helpful in certain cases; for example, testing is very useful when a doctor suspects a patient has a food allergy, or when he wants to find out the severity of an allergic response. The specific allergy tests you may encounter include the following:

Skin tests. Skin tests are the most common form of allergy testing. Your health care professional will use a skin test to determine the nature of your allergy, most often if you have asthma, hay fever, or *eczema.* The test works by measuring the level of IgE antibodies you secrete in response to various triggers. During a skin test, your health care professional will either inject a solution that contains different allergies under your skin (for example, dust mites, pollens, different foods, etc.), or she will apply them with a small scratch. She will then examine the area of your skin where she delivered the trigger to see if you exhibit an allergic-type response. An allergic reaction usually shows up as a small red raised area with a surrounding flush, similar to a mosquito bite.

One specific type of skin test is called a *patch test,* which is done to determine whether an allergic reaction has been caused by the skin rubbing against a certain substance, such as an earring or a dye used in clothing. A patch test is exactly what it sounds like: During the test, your doctor will place an adhesive patch containing various potentially allergenic substances on your skin for 48 to 72 hours. If you develop a small skin rash resembling poison ivy, you are indeed allergic to one of the substances.

Blood tests. Blood tests for allergies work similarly to skin tests in that they measure IgE antibodies, only they measure them directly in the blood instead of the skin. Although 400 different blood samples can be tested, your physician will choose which triggers to test for. Your physician may choose to use a blood test if you cannot get or do not want a skin test. For example, people with eczema have a hard time tolerating tests done directly on their skin. The most common blood test used for allergies is called the *radioallergosorbent test (RAST).* Other blood tests you might encounter include a test for your antibody/immunoglobulin levels (especially IgE) and a *complete blood count* (see Immune System Tests below).

Oral challenge. If a skin test fails to diagnose your suspected food or drug allergy (for instance, if your skin still indicates you have a milk allergy, but you have actually outgrown the symptoms), you may take an *oral challenge.* Oral challenge tests carry the potential for anaphylaxis, so they are done in doctors' offices or hospitals where you can get immediate care in the case of an emergency. During the test, you will get small doses of various substances, after which you will be monitored for allergy symptoms such as hives, wheezing, or a drop in blood pressure.

Use or elimination tests. In some cases, particularly if he suspects you may have a food or medication allergy, your physician may tell you to avoid certain substances or foods to see if you improve. If your reactions are not severe, he may also ask you to use some suspected items to see if you feel worse.

Double-blind food challenge. As a second step to a food elimination test, your doctor may do a *double-blind food challenge.* During this test, which is only done if your reactions are not severe, you will swallow a series of capsules containing various potential triggers one at a time, and neither you nor your doctor will know which capsule contains the substance you are allergic to. After you swallow each capsule, the doctor will watch to see if you experience a reaction. Because it is expensive, you probably won't undergo a double-blind food test unless your doctor suspects your allergic reactions are due to something other than food. Occasionally, a placebo is used and the gold standard food test is called the double-blind placebo-controlled food challenge (DBPCFC).

Immune system tests. In some cases, allergies are the result of a larger problem with the police force that guards your body from bacteria and other invaders: your immune system. If your allergy or asthma symptoms are particularly severe or hard to control, or they show up together with unusual infections, an immune system abnormality may be to blame. The catchall test of the immune system is the complete blood count, which measures your white blood cell count, your platelets (substances in your blood that help it clot), and your hematocrit (the concentration of your blood). This test can be broken down further to look at levels of specific white blood cells, including lymphocytes, neutrophils, eosinophils, and basophils. Another common test involves measuring immunoglobulin levels (IgG, IgA, IgM, and IgE).

Peak flow measurement. If you suffer from asthma, *peak flow measurement* is one of the simplest and most useful tests, and you can also take it at home. To perform the test, you blow into a handheld device that gives you a reading called a peak flow rate, usually given in liters per minute. If you perform a peak flow measurement test daily, you will get a warning of when an asthma attack is coming so you can contact your doctor.

Pulmonary function test. Another asthma test, the *pulmonary function test* (also called spirometry) is often used to make a definite diagnosis of asthma. To do the test, you will blow into a machine that measures your breathing before and after you use an inhaler. If your breathing improves after using the inhaler, you probably indeed have asthma.

Chest X ray. To rule out diseases such as pneumonia or a sinus disease that may be causing your symptoms, your doctor may order a *chest X ray.* Chest X rays are quick and painless—you will receive a small amount of radiation for just a few minutes.

CT (CAT) scan. To rule out a chronic sinus problem, a *CT scan* creates a detailed image of your sinuses. This test is usually done in less than 15 minutes and is also painless.

Sweat test. If your allergy symptoms include breathing problems associated with repeated pneumonia, digestion issues, and slowed growth, your doctor will want to rule out a disease called cystic fibrosis. The test for cystic fibrosis involves getting you to sweat and then testing the salt in your secretions—high salt levels in sweat indicate you may have cystic fibrosis instead of an allergy.

pH probe test. Sometimes allergy and asthma symptoms can spring from gastroesophageal reflux disorder (GERD), a condition in which your stomach acid travels upward into your esophagus. To rule out GERD, you may have to take a *pH probe test,* which measures the stomach acid in your esophagus for 24 hours.

Echocardiogram. In some cases, wheezing, asthma, or other breathing-related reactions may be related to a problem with your heart instead of an allergy trigger. During an echocardiogram, which is painless and takes less than 30 minutes, a technician will use an ultrasound wand to create images of your heart. By looking at your heart's movements, your health care professional will be able to tell if your heart is working properly. If so, your symptoms are more likely to be caused by allergies.

Other tests. Beyond the tests listed above, your physician may check your reaction to physical triggers by stimulating you with heat or cold and watching for a reaction. He may also drop a dissolved form of the trigger into your lower eyelid and watch for a response there.

Common Diagnostic Tests for Allergies

The most common diagnostic tests for allergies include:

Skin tests: Skin tests are the most common form of allergy testing. The test works by measuring the level of IgE antibodies you secrete in response to various triggers.

Oral challenge: During an oral challenge test, you will get small doses of various substances, after which you will be monitored for allergy symptoms such as hives, wheezing, or a drop in blood pressure. Oral challenge tests carry the potential for anaphylaxis, so they are done in doctors' offices or hospitals where you can get immediate care in the case of an emergency.

Blood tests: Blood tests for allergies work similarly to skin tests in that they measure IgE antibodies, only they measure them directly in the blood instead of the skin. The most common blood test used for allergies is called the radioallergosorbent test (RAST). Other blood tests you might encounter include a test for your antibody/immunoglobulin levels (especially IgE) and a complete blood count.

Use or elimination tests: In some cases, your physician may tell you to avoid certain substances or foods to see if you improve. If your reactions are not severe, he may also ask you to use some suspected items to see if you feel worse.

Peak flow measurement: If you suffer from asthma, you will most likely take a peak flow measurement test. To perform the test, you blow into a handheld device that gives you a reading called a peak flow rate, usually given in liters per minute.

WHAT YOU NEED TO KNOW

▸ Many people think they have allergies to things like cigarette smoke, paint fumes, perfumes and other strong smells, plastics, and temperature changes, when in fact they have nonallergic reactions to these things and not true allergies. Only a medical doctor can make a definitive allergy diagnosis.

▸ Similarly, many people falsely think they have food allergies to things such as milk, gluten, and MSG, when in fact they have intolerances or sensitivities to these foods.

▸ People with allergies often develop asthma, which involves coughing, wheezing, and shortness of breath as a result of narrowing airways in the lungs.

▸ Allergies that produce sneezing and a runny nose can transition into more painful and dangerous sinusitis.

▸ You can see your family doctor or an allergist for your allergies, but an allergist has more training in the area of allergies and therefore is likely to have a better-targeted approach.

3

Allergy Triggers

About a month after she started her summer job as a vet technician, Julia, age 18, thought she might have to quit. Every day, soon after she arrived at the veterinarian's office, she was crippled by itchy, red, watery eyes, a runny nose, and sneezing and coughing fits. Julia was convinced she was allergic to the dogs, cats, and other pets she loved working with so much, but a trip to the allergist revealed that it wasn't the cute furry creatures that were making Julia's life at her summer job so miserable—it was the latex gloves she had to put on to do the less pleasant parts of her job. Upon learning about the true cause of her allergy, Julia was able to keep her job by switching to latex-free gloves. Now, as long as she stays away from natural latex, Julia can happily and ably clip nails, draw blood, and cuddle with each pet she sees.

Julia's story is a prime example of why it is so important for teens with allergies to be aware of the substances that may be triggering their symptoms. We're all quick to point the finger at pollen and dust because many people are allergic to these things; but there are actually more than 240 different allergens out there, including vanilla, lentils, pigeons, silk, and numerous other substances you might never suspect. These allergens can cause a range of reactions, including asthma, stomach problems, hay fever, skin reactions, watery eyes, anaphylaxis, and more. The more you know about allergy triggers and the symptoms they cause, the better you and your physician will be able to correctly identify the real root of the problem. Here are some allergy triggers and their symptoms for your review.

POLLEN

If you sniffle and sneeze at certain times of the year only, you probably have an allergy to some kind of pollen. Pollens are tiny, egg-shaped male cells of flowering plants. Although they are small—no wider than the average human hair—they can pack a big wallop when it comes to allergies. You may be tempted to point the finger at rosebushes, peonies, or other brightly colored flowers as the cause of your sniffles, but the pollens from these prettier plants usually don't trigger allergies. It's either the trees in your backyard, the grasses in the nearby field, or the weeds cropping up in your garden that are actually to blame.

Pollens wreak such havoc on people who are allergic to them in part because millions—sometimes billions—of particles are released by a single plant, and these particles can travel for up to 200 miles. Therefore, if you have a pollen allergy, you will be affected not only by the plants in your backyard, but also by plants growing across the state as well. Between August and September alone, an estimated 300 million tons of pollen are circulated through the air. Pollens are like tiny balloons that float through the air together in bunches, and although you may think it is yellow pollen you see on the car windshield or windowsill that's making you sneeze, it is more often the colorless pollen that's the problem. Because insects can't see the transparent pollens, they don't use them for fertilization, and therefore there is more of this type left floating in the air and into your eyes and nostrils.

Symptoms of pollen allergies include a runny nose, sneezing, congestion, itchy, watery eyes, and an itchy throat, roof of your mouth, or ears. Together, these symptoms are called hay fever.

Contrary to popular belief, pollens don't only strike people in the spring; just like holiday decorations, different types of pollens come out at different times of the year . . . only they don't bring happiness and cheer. Allergies that start in April and May are usually due to pollens from trees such as oak, western red cedar, elm, ash, birch, hickory, maple, sycamore, and walnut. Summer allergies in late May through July are usually the result of pollens from grasses and weeds such as timothy, orchard, sweet vernal, red top, Bermuda, and some blue grasses. Fall allergies from late August through the first frost are most often due to *ragweed*, pigweed, tumbleweed, sagebrush, cockleweed, and Russian thistle.

What's more, weather can make your pollen allergy better or worse. When it's rainy, cloudy, or windless, you will probably feel better because pollen can't travel very far in these conditions. If it's

Pollen and Mold Counts

It may seem like just a number, but if you are allergic, a pollen or mold count can make a huge difference in how you feel. So these are numbers you are going to want to pay attention to.

Just like the weather, pollen and mold counts change daily based on the time of year, where you live in the country, and other factors. Interpretations of pollen and mold counts are fairly complex. Factors can interfere with the numbers, including the device used and its location. The counts are reported as grains per cubic meter of air—naturally, more grains equal more discomfort for you. Most people develop symptoms when pollen counts reach 20 to 100 grains per cubic meter, but this is not an exact science; your individual sensitivity and whether or not you were exposed to pollen in the days preceding the count also interfere.

You can get these counts by going to your local university, medical center, or clinic, or by simply jumping on the Internet. As a free service to the public, the National Allergy Bureau (NAB) compiles pollen and mold counts as reported by certified stations across the country and announces them each week on the NAB page of the American Academy of Allergy, Asthma and Immunology's Web site at http://www.aaaai.org.

hot, dry, and windy, on the other hand, you will probably feel your allergy symptoms more severely and therefore not be able to enjoy the sunny weather quite as much as your nonallergic friends.

MOLDS

Molds are microscopic fungi that live off of decaying plant life. Anywhere water tends to collect, such as damp basements, shower curtains, rotting logs, hay, mulch, basements, refrigerators, garbage cans, and window moldings, you can find mold. Naturally, mold is worse when the weather is damp or rainy. Molds give off spores that can float through the air like pollen. When those spores reach someone who is allergic to them, they trigger symptoms. Unfortunately, however, molds do not have a specific season, so they can plague you at any time of the year if you live in the Southern or Western states. In other areas, molds peak in July in warmer states and October in colder states. Dying vegetation in the fall, such as piles of leaves, are loaded with mold.

If you have a mold allergy, you will feel worse when the weather is damp, and you will notice symptoms when you are in a musty basement or near hay straw, wet leaves, or a compost pile. Symptoms of mold allergies are similar to those of pollen allergies and include congestion, sneezing, runny nose, coughing, itchy, watery eyes, and, in severe cases, asthma.

INSECT BITES AND STINGS

The venom that an insect injects into you when it bites or stings causes an allergic reaction in some people far more annoying than the initial burning pain of the attack. All people will react to an insect bite or sting in some way. People who are not allergic will have pain, swelling and redness in the area. In others, it can be severe enough to be fatal. The five most common insects whose stings cause allergic reactions are yellow jackets, honeybees, paper wasps, hornets, and fire ants.

In people who are allergic to insect bites and stings, their immune systems overreact to the venom. After the first sting—for example, by a yellow jacket—an allergic person's body produces the allergic substance immunoglobulin E (IgE) antibody, which reacts with the venom. Then the next time that person is stung by a yellow jacket, the venom will interact with the IgE once again, this time triggering the release of histamine among other mediators and all the nasty symptoms that go along with it. Some people with milder insect bite and sting allergies will suffer swelling that goes beyond the sting site; for example, someone who is stung in the forearm may have swelling that causes his arm to be twice its normal size. People with severe allergies to insect bites and stings, however, may experience a life-threatening reaction called anaphylaxis. Symptoms of anaphylaxis include swelling of the throat or tongue, trouble breathing, hives, dizziness, stomach cramps, nausea, diarrhea, low blood pressure, and loss of consciousness. People who suffer anaphylaxis after an insect sting must carry a dosage of medicine whenever there is a chance they might encounter the insect they are allergic to. If they are stung, emergency medical care is often necessary.

To avoid the five most common allergy-triggering insects, you must first know what they look like.

Yellow jackets are black and yellow, and their nests are usually located underground or in the walls of frame buildings, wood piles, or cracks in stones or concrete.

Honeybees have dark brown and yellow round fuzzy bodies, and they live in honeycombs in hollow trees or holes in buildings.

Paper wasps have long, skinny bodies that are brown, black, or red and yellow. They're called paper wasps because of the paper-like nests they build in woodpiles, in shrubs, or behind shutters.

Hornets are black or brown with orange, yellow, or white markings and legs that dangle when they fly. Their nests are brown or gray and shaped like a football and usually found in high places like tree hollows or branches.

Fire ants are reddish colored ants related to bees. They build tall nests (up to 18 inches high) in the ground. A fire ant stings by gripping the victim's skin by its teeth, arching its back and pivoting its head to create a burning sensation.

FOODS

There is a chapter devoted completely to food allergies later in this book, but here is a preview: The most common food allergy triggers are peanuts, tree nuts, eggs, wheat, soy, shellfish, fish, and dairy products. Although 13 to 18 percent of the population *think* they have food allergies, only about two percent actually do. With that being said, however, seven million Americans have real food allergies, three million of which are the most serious kinds—peanut and tree nut allergies, which cause anaphylaxis.

Food allergies are most common in infants and often go away as a person gets older. Peanut allergies are the exception, however—only 10 to 20 percent of people lose their peanut allergies in adulthood as compared to 90 percent of people with other food allergies. Allergists describe the "allergic arch," where as food allergies decline in toddlers, airborne allergies come to the fore. With the exception of anaphylaxis-inducing peanut and tree nut allergies, most food allergies cause annoying symptoms such as a stuffy nose, swollen lips, wheezing, stomach cramps, vomiting, diarrhea, hives, eczema, or an itchy rash.

MEDICATIONS

Ironically, some medicines you take to feel better can actually make you feel much worse, and this is definitely the case for any medications you are allergic to. Prescription medications used to treat infections—called antibiotics—cause allergic reactions more often than any other type of drug. If you've ever been asked if you are allergic to penicillin, for example, your doctor was referring to a type of antibiotic that is well known for causing allergies. Other medications that can cause allergic reactions include insulin, local anesthetics, dyes injected for X-rays, and classes of medications called sulphas and barbiturates.

Drug allergies are rare, but when they do strike they can cause a range of reactions from mild to moderate itching, hives, rashes, headaches, and nausea to life-threatening anaphylaxis that involves allover itchiness, swelling of the face and throat, increased heart rate, trouble breathing, and loss of consciousness. Other symptoms of drug allergies include asthma and sinus, eye, and ear irritation. Allergic reactions to medications may strike right away or take a few hours to set in.

DUST MITES

Dust mites are tiny critters that can be found anywhere there is dust—in bedding, mattresses, upholstered furniture, and carpeting. A relative of the spider, the dust mite also has eight legs, but it is microscopic—as many as 19,000 dust mites may live in one gram of dust (a gram of dust is about the size of a paper clip). There are two different species of house dust mites in North America. They feed on human skin scales, fungi, bacteria, pollen, and animal dander. Dust mites love moisture, so they do best in humidity levels of 70 to 80 percent. One study showed that dust mites die out when the humidity level drops below 60 percent. Each dust mite produces about 10–20 waste particles per day, which is important because people who are allergic to dust mites are actually reacting to the proteins in their feces that hide in pillows, mattresses, carpeting, and upholstered furniture. Specifically, it is the proteins on the surface of dust mites' feces that cause an allergic reaction. As disgusting as it might sound, dust mites are "coprophillic," meaning they eat their own feces and therefore continue to coat the feces with more allergenic protein. Believe it or not, the average person who is allergic to dust mites spends one-third of his life with his nose pressed up against a pillow loaded with the little buggers. Dust mites also love pet skin and dander, so there will be quite a few hanging out where your pet sleeps.

Although dust mites thrive in areas where there are people, the good news is that they do not bite, they don't burrow under the skin, and they cannot spread diseases. In fact, dust mites are only harmful to you if you are allergic to them. Symptoms of an allergy to the dust mite include itchy, watery eyes, sneezing, stuffy ears, runny nose, respiratory problems, eczema, and, in severe cases, asthma. If you have a dust mite allergy, you may notice that your symptoms get worse after you or a family member stirs up dust while cleaning. While the dust is in the air, you will inhale the tiny dust mite feces and body fragments mixed in with it. However, it may not be the dust mite parts but the dust itself that you are allergic to; you will need to see your family doctor or an allergist to get a proper diagnosis.

DUST

Where there is a dust mite, obviously, there is house dust. House dust is a mixture of lots of different things found in your home—fibers from carpeting and drapes, food remnants, pet hair, pet dander, debris from furniture, and outside dust from traffic or nearby construction sites. In many cases, a person is not allergic to dust itself but to one of the ingredients in dust, such as food particles or mold spores. The dust components that are most likely to trigger allergies include chalk/eraser dust, pieces of carpeting and rugs, drapes, upholstered furniture remnants, toys, cockroach particles, and attic or basement dust. Although you might be tempted to blame your mom, dad, or sibling (whoever last did the dusting in your house) for their poor cleaning skills, you can hold your breath. Normal housecleaning may not be enough to remove dust from your home.

Symptoms of dust allergy mimic those of other common allergies and include runny or stuffy nose, sneezing, and itchy, watery eyes. If you have asthma, you may also experience wheezing, coughing, and shortness of breath in response to dust.

COCKROACHES

Cockroaches are beetly-looking bugs with long antennas and a hard shell. These bugs are surprisingly adaptable; in fact, they have existed in their current form for 400 million years. (So they probably roamed with the dinosaurs at some point in time!) These bugs can live anywhere at any time of year and if they can find food, warmth, and moisture, they will stay. The cockroach's favorite places to hide (in this order) are: kitchen cabinets, kitchen floors, damp basements, mattresses, upholstered furniture, bathrooms, soft furnishings, toilets, and bedrooms. Although for most people they are certainly not pretty to look at, cockroaches are actually fairly harmless, unless you are allergic to their bodily waste. Similarly to a dust mite, cockroach waste triggers allergic reactions in some people.

An estimated 10 million people in the United States are allergic to cockroaches, and about 40 percent of people with asthma are thought to have the allergy. Symptoms of cockroach allergy include itchy and watery eyes, sneezing, congestion, and/or asthma.

LATEX

When Julia experienced the runny nose, sneezing, and other discomforts after putting on latex gloves, her body's immune system was reacting to the proteins in the rubber latex. If you have experienced a similar reaction to Julia's after coming in contact with balloons, latex gloves, or other latex products, you too may have a latex allergy. One to 6 percent of the general population has sensitivities to latex, compared with up to 10 percent of people who work in the health-care industry, indicating that latex allergies may develop after a person has been exposed to latex for a while.

Latex is produced from a natural rubber plant, more specifically, the sap of a tree called the *Hevea braziliensis* that's found in Africa and Southeast Asia. Natural rubber latex should not be confused with petroleum or butyl-based synthetic rubber products. The latex products that most frequently cause allergy symptoms include balloons, rubber toys, rubber bands, baby bottle nipples and pacifiers, condoms, diapers, sanitary pads, and adhesive tape and bandages. Synthetic products such as latex house paints do not appear to cause symptoms in people with latex allergies.

It's not surprising that Julia attributed her allergies to animals because symptoms of latex allergies mimic those of other allergies, including allergies to pets. Latex allergies can build up over time, becoming more severe each time the person is exposed to the rubber; or, they can strike at a life-threatening level with no previous symptoms or warning signs. Symptoms usually develop within 12 to 36 hours after exposure to latex and include itchy, red, watery eyes, sneezing, runny nose, coughing, hives or skin rash, cracked, red, raised areas on skin that was exposed to latex, and shortness of breath and chest tightness. In severe cases, the person may even go into shock.

ANIMALS

It is also not surprising that Julia first blamed the animals in the vet's office for her allergies because animals are one of the most common allergy triggers, especially cats. An estimated 10 percent of the population is allergic to animals, and 20 to 30 percent of people with asthma have animal allergies. However, it's not the animals them-selves, but the proteins found on their skin and in their saliva and urine that cause the sniffles and sneezing. You can expose yourself to these proteins by holding an animal, being in the same room with an animal, or by simply coming into contact with dust that contains an animal's dander—even when that animal is nowhere to be found.

Pet Allergies

Pets make a wonderful addition to the family. They provide security, companionship, and joy, and children often learn valuable lessons about responsibility from them. So it's no wonder that there are 100,000,000 pets in this country and more than 70 percent of U.S. households have a dog or cat. Unfortunately, 10 percent of the population is allergic to pets, so there is bound to be crossover between the pet owners and the pet allergies. The most common household pets are dogs, cats, birds, hamsters, rabbits, mice, gerbils, rats, and guinea pigs, all of which can cause allergies. Contrary to popular belief, short haired animals do not cause fewer problems—people are allergic to pets' dander and the proteins in their saliva and urine, not their hair. Animal allergies can take two or more years to develop, long after you and your family members have gotten attached to Fido or Fluffy, and allergies often don't subside until months after your pet has left the home, so you will probably not get immediate relief once they are out. Symptoms of *pet allergies* include sneezing, itchy, watery eyes, and congestion.

A good test to see whether or not you are allergic to your pet is to monitor your symptoms when you are on vacation or visiting a friend—away from your pet—for two to three weeks. If you feel better when your dog, cat, or other pet is not around, he or she is probably the culprit.

The best way to get rid of pet allergies is to get rid of the pet that is causing them or move the pet outside or at least from the bedroom. This is not an acceptable solution for some people, however. In that case, you can try medications such as antihistamines, *decongestants,* nasal *steroids,* or *immunotherapy.* When all else fails, the best pet for an allergic individual is a tropical fish in a small aquarium (larger aquariums can add moisture and mold to the house).

Also, it takes a few months for the allergy to develop. One patient got a kitten for Christmas and developed allergy symptoms in May—no surprise since animal allergies typically take four to six months to develop. Beyond live animals, your mom's cashmere sweater or mohair scarf may cause the problem, as can down comforters and horsehair-stuffed chairs and couches.

Symptoms of animal allergies include wheezing; sneezing; coughing; itchy, watery, and swollen eyes; itchy, runny nose; congestion; shortness of breath; and in severe cases, a rash on the face, neck, and upper chest.

INDOOR AIR POLLUTION

Ironically, the things we use to make our homes smell fresh and clean—bath oils, cleaning products, scented candles, insect repellants, and floor waxes—can trigger allergies. If your home is ventilated poorly, it only makes things worse. Cigarette smoke and other tobacco smoke are common indoor allergens. Studies have shown that children exposed to tobacco smoke—even when only one parent smokes—have an increased risk of developing allergies and respiratory infections, whether they have allergies or not. Other common indoor allergens include:

- natural gas
- cosmetics
- glue
- ammonia
- perfumes
- gasoline
- motor oil
- nail polish
- detergents

OUTDOOR AIR POLLUTION

Smog, the heavy, gray cloud of air pollution that hangs over most major cities, is not only an eyesore on otherwise pretty skylines; it can trigger allergies. In big cities, heavy traffic and industries create a cloud of ozone, nitrogen dioxide, and petroleum-produced chemicals called hydrocarbons. Warm and sunny cities like Los Angeles and Miami have particularly severe smog problems. In sensitive people, smog can cause breathing problems, eye irritation, tiredness, and other symptoms.

CHEMICALS

If you have ever broken out in hives or a rash after mom switched to a new fabric softener or you decided to buy a new concealer that was on sale to hide a pimple, you may have had a reaction to the chemicals used in these products. Dyes in your clothing, household cleaners, and pesticides sprayed on your lawn or inside your home can also trigger an irritating reaction, usually in the form of a skin rash. This reaction is not technically an allergy, however.

OTHER ALLERGIES

As odd as it may sound, some people are sensitive to hot or cold temperatures, sunlight, or other everyday physical stimuli. In some, simply rubbing their skin will cause a reaction. However, these reactions are not true allergies because people do not develop an IgE antibody to them. Even if you think you have your allergy pinned, the only way to know for sure what you are allergic to and to get proper treatment is to get a firm diagnosis from a health care professional.

THE TOP 10 SKIN ALLERGENS

One of the most common allergic reactions is that which occurs on the skin. If you are susceptible to an allergic reaction on the skin known as contact dermatitis, chances are it doesn't take much to set your skin off. You have probably reacted to jewelry, lotions, perfumes, colognes, and more, but if you know what can produce a reaction, you can better prevent your skin from becoming swollen, itchy, and red. Here is a list of the top 10 skin allergens, compiled by a team of experts at the Mayo Clinic after they tested 69 different allergens on 3,854 patients:

- **Nickel,** a metal frequently used in jewelry (particularly, plated white gold), jewelry clasps, and buttons on clothing
- **Gold** jewelry
- **Formaldehyde,** a preservative used in household cleaners, cosmetics, medications, paints, and paper products
- A tree-resin derived fragrance used in perfumes and skin lotions called **Balsam of Peru**
- **Fragrance mix,** a group of the eight most frequently used fragrance allergens in cosmetics, soaps, foods, perfumes, antiseptics, dental products, and insecticides

‣ **Cobalt chloride,** a metal used in some hair dyes, antiperspirants, metal-plated objects, such as buttons, snaps, and tools, and in cobalt blue pigments
‣ **Quaternium 15,** a preservative used in some beauty products such as shampoo, nail polish, self-tanners, sunscreens, as well as in some industrial paints, polishes, and waxes
‣ **Bacitracin,** a topical antibiotic
‣ **Thimerosal,** a mercury compound found in vaccines and local antiseptics
‣ **Neomycin sulfate,** a topical antibiotic commonly found in first aid ointments and occasionally in deodorant, soap, makeup, and pet food

WHAT YOU NEED TO KNOW

‣ As a free service to the public, the National Allergy Bureau (NAB) compiles pollen and mold counts as reported by certified stations across the country and announces them each week on the NAB page of The American Academy of Allergy, Asthma and Immunology's Web site at http://www.aaaai.org.
‣ People with severe allergies to insect bites and stings, foods, or drugs may experience a life-threatening reaction called anaphylaxis. Symptoms of anaphylaxis include swelling of the throat or tongue, trouble breathing, hives, dizziness, stomach cramps, nausea, diarrhea, low blood pressure, and loss of consciousness.
‣ Seven million Americans have real food allergies, three million of which are the most serious kinds—peanut and tree nut allergies, which cause anaphylaxis.
‣ With the exception of anaphylaxis-inducing peanut and tree nut allergies, most food allergies cause annoying symptoms such as a stuffy nose, swollen lips, wheezing, stomach cramps, vomiting, diarrhea, hives, eczema, or an itchy rash.
‣ Drug allergies are rare, but when they do strike they can cause a range of reactions from mild to moderate itching, hives, rashes, headaches, and nausea to life-threatening anaphylaxis that involves allover itchiness, swelling of the face and throat, increased heart rate, trouble breathing, and loss of consciousness.
‣ An estimated 10 million people in the United States are allergic to cockroaches, and about 40 percent of people with asthma are thought to have the allergy.

➤ The best way to get rid of pet allergies is to get rid of the pet that is causing them or to move the pet outside or at least from the bedroom.
➤ Smog, the heavy, gray cloud of air pollution that hangs over most major cities, is not only an eyesore on otherwise pretty skylines; it can trigger allergies.

4

Fighting Back:
Allergy Medications

Every summer for most of her childhood, Lauren, now age 16, sat by the community pool with tissues in hand. For her, June meant the end of school and the beginning of summer fun, but it also meant the start of severe allergy symptoms that got in the way of fun at camp, water parks, and the beach. When Lauren reached age 12, her symptoms got even worse, and she decided she had suffered through her last summer. Under her doctor's advice, Lauren started allergy shots. Four years later, she views the start of summer with a whole new attitude. Instead of taking the good times with the bad allergies, she enjoys sunning, swimming, and other outdoor activities allergy-free. For Lauren, a few seconds of discomfort from the occasional shots have made a huge difference in her life.

If you suffer from allergies or asthma, chances are you, like Lauren, will take a medication to ease your symptoms at one time or another. If your allergies are severe, you will probably take medications frequently, possibly in the form of allergy shots. If your allergies are mild, you might only take medications now and then.

Unfortunately, there are no magic pills for allergies. No medications can cure an allergy completely, and different drugs work well in different people. What medications can do, however, is reduce the discomfort that allergies cause so you can camp, go swimming, shop, and ride your bike with your friends without worrying about sniffling, sneezing, or running frantically from a bee. In short, like they did for Lauren, allergy medications can improve your life.

Allergies and asthma are different from other medical conditions for which you take medication in that there is no one straightforward, cookie-cutter approach. Let's take acne, for example. If you have a chronic acne problem, you may take antibiotics regularly to keep the pimples under control. Your doctor may try several different drugs until he finds the right one for you, but he will only try one medication at a time—you would never take them all at once.

The treatment of allergies is more complicated. Often, multiple medications are prescribed at the same time to attack different aspects of the allergy in various parts of your body. Some allergy medications block the release of chemicals that cause allergic reactions, some reduce swelling, some stop muscle constriction, and some fight inflammation. On the one hand, this is a good thing—it means that allergists are better than ever at prescribing the right medications to target precise allergy symptoms, so that no unrelated tissues get damaged. On the other hand, it means more responsibility on the part of the person taking the medications. Because of their specificity, allergy medications require a strict adherence to dosages and timetables. That's why it is so important for you to clearly understand the medications you take for your allergies. The more you know about them and the better you understand how they work, the better they will serve you. The following overview will help.

There are many effective medications available to control allergies, and your doctor can help you identify the one or ones that will work best for you depending on the type and severity of your symptoms and the medications' side effects. The most common types and forms of medications used in the treatment of allergies are antihistamines, decongestants, antihistamine and decongestant combinations, anti-inflammatory medications, immunotherapy (allergy shots), *nasal sprays, bronchodilators,* and emergency medications. In addition to the medications covered below, there are many other drugs available. Your doctor can help you choose the best medications for you.

ANTIHISTAMINES

The most popular of the allergy medications—antihistamines—work to prevent or relieve the effects of the substance histamine, including sneezing, itching, watery eyes, runny nose, and difficulty breathing. When you encounter an allergen, your cells produce histamine, along with cytokines and leukotrienes, in response to IgE antibodies. This histamine is what causes the annoying reaction in your eyes, nose, throat, lungs, skin, or intestinal tract. Antihistamines, as their name suggests, block the ill effects of histamine. These medications are most effective if you take them prior to being exposed to an allergen; for example, before a trip to an animal shelter or an open field.

You can buy some antihistamines over the counter at your local drugstore, and others are available only with a doctor's prescription. Over-the-counter (OTC) antihistamines include Allegra, *Benadryl, Claritin, Chlor-Trimeton, Dimetane, Tavist,* and Zyrtec. These OTC antihistamines range from short-acting—meaning they help relieve mild to moderate allergy symptoms—to longer-acting versions that are generally stronger and prescribed for more severe allergies (*fexofenadine* [Allegra] and *cetirizine* [Zyrtec]).

In addition to being the most commonly used, antihistamines are among the oldest remedies for allergies. For generations, people have been using antihistamines to ease allergy symptoms, and these medicines have gotten more effective over the years. The older formulas—Benadryl, Chlor-Trimeton, and Dimetapp—caused severe drowsiness, worked for only six hours, and required additional decongestants to relieve stuffiness. Newer formulas, such as the recently introduced *levocetirizine* (Xysal), relieve allergy symptoms and improve overall quality of life without additional decongestants.

In addition to the oral pill and liquid forms, antihistamines are available in nasal sprays and eyedrops, which are particularly effective in treating eye symptoms of allergies, including itching, watering, burning, and redness.

Antihistamines are also occasionally used to treat conditions other than allergies, for example to help prevent nausea, vomiting, and dizziness, to decrease stiffness and tremors in people with Parkinson's disease, and to relieve urticaria, a hive-like rash.

Before you take antihistamines or other allergy medications, either over-the-counter or prescription, you should talk to your doctor. Specifically, tell him or her if you have ever had an allergic or unusual reaction to an antihistamine or if you are allergic or sensitive to any other substances, such as preservatives, dyes, or foods. In addition, be sure to tell your doctor if you are on a low-sodium, low-sugar, or other special diet because most medications contain ingredients other than the active ones, such as sugar, salt, or alcohol. You should also let your doctor know if you have any medical problems that may interfere with the antihistamine, including difficulty urinating, intestinal problems, a stomach ulcer, or liver or kidney disease.

DECONGESTANTS

Another form of medication commonly used to relieve the nasal and sinus congestion that goes along with hay fever and other inhaled allergies is a decongestant. Decongestants work to help the nasal passages drain and to relieve congestion, swelling, secretions, and overall discomfort in the nose.

Decongestants are available both over-the-counter and with a prescription, and they come in pill, syrup, and nasal spray forms. OTC forms include *Sudafed* tablets or liquid, *Neo-Synephrine* and *Afrin* nasal sprays, and Visine eye drops. Prescription decongestants include *loratadine/pseudoephedrine sulfate* (Claritin-D), *fexofenadine HCl* (Allegra-D), and *cetirizine HCl* (Zyrtec-D) and combine a decongestant with another allergy medication. (If you see a *D* after the name of a medication, it means that drug contains the decongestant *pseudoephedrine*). The most popular OTC decongestant is Sudafed. However, most pharmacies keep all medications with pseudoephedrine behind the counter these days, so you may have to ask for it. Even if you choose to get the OTC form yourself, you should still discuss it with your doctor because the frequently used decongestant pseudoephedrine can have some unpleasant side effects, including nervousness, restlessness, trouble sleeping, dizziness, headache, pounding heartbeat, nausea, vomiting, and, in rare cases, convulsions. Some of these side effects can be very serious and even fatal in some cases; if you experience sudden dizziness, a fast, pounding heartbeat, severe headache, severe nausea and vomiting, or convulsions, stop taking pseudoephedrine and call your doctor right away.

ANTIHISTAMINE AND DECONGESTANT COMBINATIONS

If you have tissues spilling out of every pocket during allergy season, you may benefit from an antihistamine-decongestant combination. These medications target allergies by blocking histamine, and they also treat the runny nose, nasal congestion, and sneezing that accompany some allergies (usually hay fever). More specifically, the decongestants in these combinations work to narrow blood vessels, which helps stop your nose from running.

Just like standard antihistamines, *antihistamine-decongestant combinations* are available, depending on their strength, both over-the-counter and with a prescription from your doctor. OTC formulas include Benadryl Allergy and Sinus and Tylenol Allergy and Sinus. Prescription combinations include fexofenadine HCl (Allegra-D), loratadine/pseudoephedrine sulfate (Claritin-D), *acrivastine and pseudoephedrine* (Semprex-D), and cetirizine HCl (Zyrtec-D) for nasal allergies, and *naphazoline hydrochloride* (Naphcon, Vasocon) and *ketotifen fumarate* (Zaditor) for allergic conjunctivitis. Keep in mind that antihistamine-decongestant combinations contain ingredients that may be harmful to some people. Before you take either a prescription or OTC formula, tell your doctor if you have any allergies to medications or if you have any other medical problems, including type II diabetes, heart problems, kidney or liver disease, urinary problems, or a problem with your thyroid.

ANTI-INFLAMMATORY DRUGS

When you have a headache, anti-inflammatory drugs work to reduce the inflammation and pain in your head. When it comes to allergies, anti-inflammatory drugs, which are available both over-the-counter and with a prescription, reduce inflammation in your nose and airways, thus relieving your symptoms.

The most popular anti-inflammatory OTC medication for the treatment of allergy symptoms is *cromolyn sodium* (Intal). Cromolyn sodium is a type of medicine called a mast cell stabilizer. When mast cells in the nose encounter an allergen, they release histamine, which unleashes sniffling, sneezing, and other allergy symptoms. Cromolyn sodium and other mast cell stabilizers prevent the mast cells from releasing histamine in the first place, so you never experience the annoying symptoms.

In addition to treating runny nose, sneezing, and other symptoms of allergic rhinitis, cromolyn sodium also helps prevent the wheezing, shortness of breath, and trouble breathing caused by an allergy attack. Cromolyn sodium is available in powder-filled capsules, an inhaler, or a nasal spray.

If you know you are going to encounter an allergen, your doctor will tell you to start taking cromolyn sodium ahead of time to prevent the reaction before it has a chance to start. For example, if you are allergic to cats and you're planning a trip to visit your grandmother—who has three cats—you may want to start taking or puffing cromolyn sodium two to three days prior to build it up in your system. If you don't have that much notice, you can also take cromolyn sodium to reduce your sneezing, nasal congestion, runny nose, and eye irritation as soon as the first cat rubs against your leg. You should take cromolyn sodium for two to three days after the animal exposure is over as well.

Another class of anti-inflammatory drugs for the treatment of allergy symptoms are corticosteroids. Corticosteroids help reduce the inflammation, stuffiness, runny nose, sneezing, and itching due to both seasonal and year-round allergies. They can also reduce swelling and inflammation from other types of allergic reactions. Corticosteroids come in a number of forms, depending on the type of allergy they are being used to treat. For serious allergies or asthma, they are available in pill form. For asthma, they are offered in an inhaler. For seasonal or year-round allergies, they come in nasal sprays. For skin allergies, they are available in creams, and for allergic conjunctivitis (eye inflammation), they are available in eyedrops. Your doctor may prescribe a corticosteroid by itself or together with another allergy medication.

Corticosteroids are very effective, but you have to take them every day, even when you are not having symptoms, and it may take a week or two before the medication kicks in and starts to make you feel better. Short-term side effects of corticosteroids consist of weight gain, fluid retention, and high blood pressure. Side effects of long-term use include diabetes, muscle weakness, and osteoporosis.

Specific corticosteroid medications include the following: nasal sprays, used to treat nasal symptoms (*Nasonex, Nasocort, Beconase, Rhinocort, Flonase*); inhaled corticosteroids, used to treat asthma (*Flovent,* Azmacort, *Symbicort, Pulmicort,* and Beclovent); eyedrop forms of corticosteroids, used to treat itchy, watery eyes (*dexamethasone* [Tobradex] and *loteprednol* [Alrex]); and an oral form (*prednisone*), used to treat severe allergic reactions. For short-term skin allergies, your doctor may prescribe a topical or oral steroid cream. These are not usually prescribed for long-term skin allergies, however, because they can cause unpleasant side effects such as thinning and spotting on the skin, acne, and stretch marks.

IMMUNOTHERAPY

No one likes a needle in the arm, but if your allergies are severe enough, an occasional shot may be well worth its return in relief. Although allergy shots (called *allergen immunotherapy* in more scientific terms) are not for everyone, they help some people become steadily more tolerant of the things they are allergic to, so they can live freer, happier, less restricted lives.

Immunotherapy consists of a series of injections. These shots contain increasing concentrations of allergens over a period of time and, put simply, they work to shift the immune system. Allergy shots reduce the amount of antibodies to the allergen in your blood, which causes your body to produce a different protective antibody. Although they do not cure allergies, allergy shots tend to raise your tolerance when you are exposed to an allergen, which eases your symptoms.

Allergy shots work quite well for some people who suffer from allergies to things they breathe in (such as pollens, dust mites, cat dander) and *Hymenoptera* (bees, yellow jackets, etc.). Although you might find the idea of allergy shots unsettling, you will probably get used to them quickly (most people do), and they may do wonders for how you feel. Many people who receive allergy shots for hay fever, for example, have a less severe reaction to pollen and are able to reduce their medication within a year of starting the therapy. Studies have also shown that allergy shots are also effective if you have allergic conjunctivitis (eye irritation), an allergy to insect bites, and for some cases of allergic asthma. People who do well with allergy shots often continue them for three to four years and then stop to see if their allergies stay under control. Some are able to stop the shots indefinitely at that point, and others have to start them once again because their symptoms get worse in their absence.

The Science of Immunotherapy

Just like phones have gone from the wall to cordless to wireless, many allergy remedies have changed over the years, and numerous new drugs have been introduced, but there is nothing radically new about immunotherapy (allergy shots). People have been getting injections to help treat their allergies and asthma for almost a century. Similar to a vaccine, an allergy shot gives you a small dose of the substance to which you are allergic. Common allergies treated with allergy shots include those to weeds, mold, pollen, grasses, dust mites, household pets, and trees. (In some people, allergy shots also help treat asthma symptoms.) So if you are allergic to tree pollen, for example, your allergy shot will contain a small amount of that specific pollen.

It may seem odd to fight an allergy with the thing that causes it, but these shots alter the immune system and make it more effective at fighting the allergen the next time around. Allergy shots are usually given in gradually increasing doses. Your first shot will contain a fraction of a unit of pollen, and that dose will go up until it reaches the maximum maintenance dose. As the dose rises, you will feel better and better. The number of allergy shots you receive and the length of time you receive them will vary depending on your allergy and the way your body responds to the shots. Recent research on grass pollen, for example, shows that it takes a minimum of three years to produce an antiallergy state, and that state lasts for three or more years after the shots stop.

NASAL SPRAYS

If dust, pollen, or other airborne allergens plague you, you may benefit from a nasal spray, especially if oral antihistamines don't do the trick. Like water on a flame, nasal sprays quiet the reaction in your nasal tissues after exposure to inhaled allergens, reducing the swelling and irritation so you feel less congested. Side effects of nasal sprays include stinging or burning of the nose, bad taste, runny nose or postnasal drip, headaches, or a rash. There are a few types of nasal sprays targeted to help relieve different allergic reactions:

➤ Nasal steroid sprays (also called nasal corticosteroid sprays) reduce the reaction in your nose to inhaled allergens. These nasal sprays are available with a prescription and include *mometasone* (Nasonex), *fluticasone* (Flonase), and *triamcinolone* (Nasacort AQ). Steroid sprays usually take two weeks to start working.

➤ Cromolyn sodium (NasalCrom) is a nasal spray that helps prevent allergic reactions by stopping the release of histamine from cells, so it is more effective if you use it *before* you are exposed to an allergen. Cromolyn sodium is available without a prescription. You may have to take it for two to four weeks before it starts to work.

➤ A new antihistamine nasal spray called *azelastine* (Astelin) has been approved for people with seasonal or environmental allergies. It works similarly to oral antihistamines by blocking histamine.

➤ Decongestant nasal sprays contain the active ingredient phenylephrine, which helps constrict blood vessels and shrink nasal passages, thus stopping congestion in the short term. You shouldn't use nasal spray decongestants for more than a few days, however, because they can cause a "rebound" effect that actually makes stuffiness worse. (This is called "rhinitis medicamentosa," which is Latin for "*inflammatory* reaction in the nose.") Because of this effect, people can become addicted to decongestant nasal sprays if they use them for an extended period of time. So you should listen to the advice on the package: "If symptoms persist, contact your physician."

BRONCHODILATORS

When your airways become inflamed and swollen due to an allergy or asthma attack, they go from being flexible and expandable like a balloon to hard and rigid, like a bowling ball. Bronchodilators work to transform bowling-ball-like airways back to being soft and balloon-like once again.

Bronchodilators, such as the drugs salmeterol and *albuterol,* keep your airways open by relaxing the bronchial muscles, but the treatment doesn't end there. Albuterol is a short-acting, immediate relief bronchodilator, and salmeterol is a long-acting maintenance medication. Over time, airways that repeatedly become inflamed and inflexible injure the tissues that surround them, and these damaged tissues may require additional therapy.

Bronchodilators like salmeterol are often used as what's known as an "add-on" therapy for asthma-controlling inhaled corticosteroid medications, which helps to reduce the dosage. Bronchodilators are particularly effective if you have nighttime asthma or exercise-induced asthma that comes on after physical activity.

For chronic asthma, a bronchodilator (salmeterol)/corticosteroid combination is available in a disk-shaped metered dose contraption called a "diskus" under the brand name *Advair.* Advair is available in different strengths, but only the corticosteroid strengths change; the salmeterol stays the same. The Advair diskus is easy to use—one inhalation twice a day. In addition, the drug Symbicort, which was approved in June 2007, is Budesonide (a corticosteroid) and Formuterol (a bronchodilator). Symbicort is not a diskus but a fluorocarbon-free inhaler.

EMERGENCY ALLERGY MEDICATIONS

If you have ever had a severe allergy or asthma attack—even if only once—you should be carrying emergency medicine with you at all times, and you should know how to use it. The two most common emergency medications are emergency injection kits and the bronchodilator medication albuterol (Proventil HFA and ProAir HFA).

In the case of asthma emergencies, albuterol works as a rescue medication to open up constricted airways. It also helps to control wheezing and to prevent exercise-induced asthma.

For anaphylaxis, emergency medication injection kits called auto-injectors contain a shot of epinephrine (also called adrenaline), a fast-acting medicine that helps offset an anaphylactic reaction. (Epinephrine autoinjectors are not recommended for acute asthma.) The shot comes in an easy-to-carry container shaped like a pen, and it is marketed under the brand names EpiPen and Twinject. In the event of an attack, you inject the medication into the front of your thigh, and the injection immediately relaxes your narrowed airways and raises your blood pressure by constricting your small blood vessels.

Should You Take Allergy Shots?

Although allergy shots are very effective for some people, they are not for everyone. You are a good candidate for allergy shots if:

- ▶ Your condition has been proven to be responsive to allergy shots.

- ▶ You have allergic rhinitis, allergic conjunctivitis, asthma, an allergy to insect stings or bites, or a drug allergy.

- ▶ You are dedicated. You must be ready to stick to the whole course of treatment and not stop when you get sick of the shots or you think you feel better.

You are not a good candidate for allergy shots if:

- ▶ You have severe asthma.

- ▶ You are pregnant.

- ▶ You take heart medication (unlikely in teens, but it is worth mentioning).

- ▶ You are very sensitive to the material used.

Studies show that most of the victims who die from anaphylactic attacks are older children, teens, and young adults who have a history of an anaphylactic reaction or asthma attack, so the need to carry emergency medicine cannot be stressed enough. You can only get emergency medications with your doctor's prescription. If your doctor thinks you should carry one, he or she will give you specific instructions on how to use it in the event of an allergy attack. It's not only important that *you* know how to use the device—your teachers and friends should recognize that you are carrying it and should also know how to use it if you cannot treat yourself.

In the event that you have to use emergency medicine, you should seek medical help immediately. The effects of emergency epinephrine shots wear off in 20 to 30 minutes. Plus, an estimated one in three people has a severe enough reaction to require more than a single dose. (Twinject addresses this need and provides two doses in one.) Until help arrives, you should raise your legs above your chest to increase blood flow to your heart and brain.

Beyond the medicines discussed above, there are some additional drugs you can take to treat specific types of allergies. A medication called a leukotriene inhibitor, for example, works to block leukotrienes, substances that trigger allergies, and the prescription medication *montelukast* (Singulair) helps ease the symptoms of asthma as well as both indoor and outdoor allergies. In addition, there are two FDA-approved topical medications used to treat skin eczema—*tacrolimus* (Protopic) and *pimecrolimus* (Elidel). Your doctor can help you weed through all the medications out there to find the ones that work best for you.

OTHER ALLERGY TREATMENTS

Medications are frequently prescribed for allergies, but they are not the be-all and end-all of treatments. For certain types of allergies, for example, food allergies, the best treatment is to avoid the allergen in the first place. And there are some natural remedies you can try at home (after checking with your doctor, of course). For skin eczema, you can ease symptoms with a natural remedy, such as a room temperature bath followed by a moisturizer, and the oils found in certain types of fish, including mackerel, herring, and salmon contain eicosapentaenoic acid (EPA), which helps relieve skin itchiness and inflammation. You have to eat up to two pounds of fresh fish to get enough EPA, however, so if you're not a fish eater, you can take one tablespoon of cod liver oil or four 1,000 milligram fish oil capsules a day. You can also try taking 50 milligrams of zinc per day, which helps your body metabolize fatty acids that can contribute to the condition, as well as 25,000 IU of vitamin A per day, which can help repair and renew your skin.

In addition, simply taking a multivitamin can help ease your allergy symptoms. Vitamins C and E help boost your immune system, taking away some of the immune stress that allergies can cause, and vitamin B2 (riboflavin) can combat the sore mouth and tongue that come as a side effect of antihistamines.

TAILORING AN ALLERGY PLAN TO MATCH YOUR LIFESTYLE

The most important thing to keep in mind with regard to allergy medications is that they will only be effective if you take them properly. On

The Newest Therapy Available for Allergies and Asthma

The allergy and asthma medications you take today are similar to the ones your grandparents took, but they are constantly being improved so they relieve symptoms faster and more effectively. The most cutting-edge treatment today is Xolair. Allergists have dreamt about an "anti-IgE" medication for years, and Xolair is their dream come true. IgE is a chemical that naturally occurs in the body in small amounts, but it is produced in large quantities when an allergic person encounters the substance they are allergic to. When IgE combines with allergens, chemicals are released (including histamine) that cause the swelling, inflammation, and other allergy symptoms. The first anti-IgE drug that has been approved by the FDA for allergic asthma is omalizumab (Xolair). This medication stops the antibody IgE from reacting with an allergen in the first place, so symptoms never have a chance to occur. Xolair is given in injections, and it is usually prescribed along with inhaled corticosteroids to treat asthma. It has not yet been approved for other types of allergic reactions.

days when you feel perfectly healthy, it is easy to forget the medicines that keep you that way. That is why taking medication for your allergy symptoms requires diligence and commitment.

The best way to remember to take your allergy medication is to establish a routine. Take the medicine at the same time every day and put it in a place where you cannot forget it, like next to the loaf of bread you use to make your morning toast, or beside the bag you take to school. If you *still* have trouble remembering (as many teens do), write notes to yourself on your bedroom mirror or send yourself text messages as a reminder.

As mentioned, there is no single approach to treating allergies with medication. Most medicines have strengths and weaknesses and can be used effectively alone or together with other drugs. Your allergies are unique and different from those of other teens, so your doctor will specifically tailor your medication regimen to you and your symptoms. If you take multiple allergy medications to target different symptoms, it is also important that you take the correct medications in the proper order. Some allergy medications deal with muscle constriction, some reduce inflammation, and some target histamine. It is up to you as a responsible young adult to adhere to the instructions your doctor gives you on how and when to take your medication.

WHAT YOU NEED TO KNOW

▸ The first course of allergy treatments is usually to avoid the allergen, if possible.

▸ There is no cure for allergies, but allergy medications can provide relief of symptoms.

▸ There are many effective medications available to help treat asthma, and your doctor can help you find the ones that work best for you.

▸ Allergies and asthma are more complicated to treat with medications than other conditions because they usually attack different parts of the body at different times.

▸ The major types of allergy medications include antihistamines, anti-inflammatory drugs (including corticosteroids), decongestants, and antihistamine/decongestant combinations.

▸ Allergy drugs can be administered in a number of ways—orally, by injection (allergy shots), via nasal sprays, through bronchodilators, with eye drops, and rectally.

▸ If you have an allergy that may produce an anaphylactic reaction, your doctor will most likely advise you to carry emergency medication, such as an EpiPen or Twinject, with you at all times.

▸ In addition to medications, there are some alternative therapies you can try, such as fish oil capsules and vitamins A, C, E, and B2.

Prevention: Staving Off
an Allergy Attack

When it comes to allergies, prevention is often the best treatment. If you are allergic to cats, you shouldn't sleep with four cats on your bed every night. If you are allergic to bees, you shouldn't hang around with beekeepers. And if you are allergic to peanuts, a peanut butter and jelly sandwich should not be your lunch of choice. The prevention of other types of allergies, such as those to dust and mold, for example, can be a little trickier. Because these substances are everywhere in the environment, there is only so much you can do to avoid them. In other cases, denial gets in the way. You may love your new puppy so much that you refuse to admit that she's causing you to sneeze uncontrollably each time her cute furry little body walks into the room.

The good news when it comes to allergy prevention is that you do not have to change your lifestyle drastically, and your parents don't have to invest in expensive air filtration systems in order for you to get some relief. However, there are certain preventative measures you can and should take to minimize your exposure to the thing that makes you sniffle or itch. Here are some things you and your parents can do to make your life as a teen with allergies a little easier. You can do some of these things on your own, and others will have to be done by your parent, guardian, or other family member.

DUST ALLERGY

Dust is one of the most difficult allergies to prevent because it is *everywhere.* Unless you resign to moving into a bubble, you will never be able to avoid dust completely, but there are some simple things you and your parents can do to your environment to reduce the amount of dust and, therefore, the severity of your dust allergy symptoms.

The most important room of the house to tackle is your bedroom. Because you sleep there, you spend more time in your bedroom than in any other room in the house. Here's how to make it less dusty:

▸ As soft and cozy as they are, get rid of any down pillows or quilts; they cannot be easily washed and, therefore, they harbor dust. Instead, use hypoallergenic polyester pillows and blankets that can be washed regularly without falling apart.

▸ You should wash your bedding in hot water (at least 130 degrees Fahrenheit) every seven to 10 days.

▸ Hardwood floors are much better than carpeting. All carpets and rugs trap dust, no matter if they are made of natural or synthetic fibers. Old carpeting is the worst because it creates a lot of dust due to the breakdown of its fibers. If the carpeting in your bedroom cannot be removed, it should be professionally cleaned regularly and vacuumed daily.

▸ If you have forced air ventilation in your home, a high efficiency particulate arresting (HEPA) air filter will help remove allergens from the air in your bedroom, including dust, pet dander, or mold spores. You can run a HEPA air filter all the time, as long as doors and windows are closed.

▸ They are cute and cuddly, but stuffed animals have no place in your bedroom if you are allergic to dust because they collect it.

▸ Make sure the furniture in your bedroom is made of wood, plastic, or metal. Upholstered furniture is a dust trap.

▸ Keep your bed away from any air vents in your room and avoid storing things under it. Anything under your bed will accumulate dust that you will then breathe in when you sleep. Cover air vents with cheese cloth or another safe and appropriate material.

▸ Avoid hanging blinds in your bedroom—they are like mini shelves for dust.

▸ Unfortunately, your allergies will give your parents another reason to ask you to clean your room. You should clean your room daily and give it a really thorough cleaning at least once a week to get rid of dust. Clean your floors, windowsills and frames, and tops of doors and furniture with a damp cloth. Air the room out, but keep the door of your room closed as often as possible to avoid letting in dust from the rest of your house. You should also remove unused knickknacks, books, boxes, magazines, paper, and other clutter so dust cannot collect on it.

➤ Keep your closets clean, too. Hang all your clothing in zippered garment bags to protect them from dust, and store shoes, hats, sweaters, and other garments in boxes to eliminate dust-catching surfaces.

➤ They may be visually pleasing, but any pictures you have hanging on your walls attract dust—keep them to a minimum.

Although your bedroom is most important, the same dusting rules as above should apply to the rest of your house. In addition, you and your family should do the following:

➤ Remove drapes, upholstered furniture, feather pillows, soft toys, and non-washable comforters and blankets.

➤ Mop floors often with a damp mop.

➤ Wipe surfaces with a damp cloth.

➤ Vacuum floors regularly with a vacuum that has a high-efficiency particulate air filter. Also vacuum soft furniture and curtains.

➤ Wash any carpets and upholstery you may have with benzyl benzoate or tannic acid spray.

DUST MITES ALLERGY

Allergies to dust and allergies to dust mites closely overlap because where there is dust, often there are dust mites. To get rid of dust itself, follow the tips above. For dust mites specifically, try the following:

➤ Vacuum carpets, upholstered furniture, and mattress covers often and replace your mattress at least every 10 years.

➤ Shower and wash your hair before you go to bed.

➤ Think about investing in a dust mite detection kit, which measures how effectively you are getting rid of the mites.

➤ In areas with a high dust mite concentration, such as carpets, try sprinkling "Acarasan," a dust mite powder made by Bissell.

➤ Make sure your house is kept cool. Air conditioning may be necessary in the summer months.

➤ Dust mites love mattresses, pillows (not foam), and box springs. To keep your bed mite-free, place your mattress and box spring into an allergy-barrier zippered cover and wipe the covers off frequently.

Traveling with Allergies

When you travel to different parts of the country or the world, your allergies may worsen depending on the allergens floating around in your new environment. Be sure to check the allergy forecast in the area you will be visiting. If you are planning a cruise, be sure to survey the allergy forecasts in each country you will travel to, and realize that dust mites, mold spores, and pollen are worse in tropical, damp climates.

If you suffer from allergies to dust, dust mites, or mold, you may find that your symptoms worsen when you travel by car, bus, plane, or train. To make your traveling environment as allergen-free as possible, turn on the heater or air conditioner and let them run for a few minutes before you get into your car. Keep the windows closed to keep allergens from the outside from getting in, and travel early in the morning or late at night when the air quality is at its best.

Also realize that hotel rooms and friends' houses can be full of the same allergens you try so hard to avoid at home—dust, dust mites, and mold spores. Although there is little you can do to avoid these things, you can be prepared with your allergy medications in the event that your symptoms flare up.

COCKROACH ALLERGY

Cockroaches are a big enough turnoff on their own. Add an allergy to the mix and they are downright repulsive. Unfortunately, cockroaches are not easy to get rid off, especially if you live in a city. Here are some things you and your family members can do to help drive cockroaches—and the allergies and asthma they cause—out of your home:

▸ Clean up crumbs and spills. Cockroaches are attracted to food. Period. So the fewer morsels they can find in your drawers, microwaves, cabinets, and ovens, the better. A clean kitchen is much more likely to be cockroach-free.
▸ Wash all kitchen surfaces with soapy water daily.
▸ Keep all food in tightly sealed plastic containers or jars, or in the refrigerator.

- Eat only in the kitchen and dining room. The more rooms you eat in, the more food on the floor and the bigger the draw for cockroaches.
- Wash dishes or put them in the dishwasher immediately—don't leave them in the sink. Cockroaches don't mind your leftovers, and they will seek out the food left on plates.
- Empty trash cans daily. Keep all trash in cans with lids and in plastic bags that tie at the top.
- Don't let pet food sit out. If your cat or dog doesn't finish it, put it away.
- Make sure all holes and cracks in your home are sealed and that leaky plumbing is repaired. To cockroaches, holes and leaks are attractive and cozy hideaways.
- Change kitty litter no less often than once every few days.
- Throw away or recycle any paper goods, such as newspapers, paper bags, and magazines that are sitting around the house, especially those that came from the grocery store. Believe it or not, grocery stores often harbor roaches, and one or two may have hitched a ride to your house in a paper grocery bag.
- Try to reduce the humidity in your house because cockroaches love moisture. If necessary, get a *dehumidifier* or, at the very least, use a fan. To discourage cockroaches, aim for 40% to 50% relative humidity.
- Remove any rotting floors or damp wallpaper.
- Use safe insecticides to help get rid of the roaches. Gel baits and bait stations are the most effective and the safest for eliminating them. Baits should go in all rooms of the house, as long as they are out of the reach of small children, and they should be changed every three months.
- Your family should avoid using insect sprays or pesticide bombs to get rid of cockroaches—they can cause asthma symptoms worse than those caused by the cockroaches themselves.

POLLEN ALLERGY

Pollen allergies are tough when it comes to prevention. Short of staying inside for the entire spring or summer, there is little you can do to avoid pollens completely. Because pollens can travel for hundreds of miles, clearing the problem trees, bushes, or weeds out of your yard does little good. Moving to a different area of the country usually doesn't help either because you will probably develop allergies to a new tree or plant in that area as well. However, there are some

What Is a Peak Flow Meter? Where Do I Get One and How Do I Use It?

A *peak flow meter* is a portable handheld device that measures your ability to push air out of your lungs. Many doctors think people with asthma can benefit from the use of peak flow meters; they give you an idea of how well your lungs are working, so you can adjust your daily asthma medication accordingly.

You can also use a peak flow meter to help you and your doctor identify the causes of your asthma at home, school, or play. In addition, it can be used during an asthma attack to help you determine the severity of the episode and decide if you should use a rescue medication, and whether or not you should seek emergency medical help. There are two types of peak flow meters—a low range meter for children, and a standard range meter for older children, teenagers like yourself, and adults. There are several types of peak flow meters available, and your doctor can tell you which one is most appropriate for you.

To use the meter, you will stand up straight, remove any gum or food from your mouth, take a deep breath, and blow into the meter by closing your lips as tightly around the mouthpiece as possible. You will repeat the routine three times to make sure the numbers come out close together. You will then record the highest of the three numbers (do not calculate an average).

things you can do to keep your pollen exposure to a minimum. Here are some suggestions:

▸ Avoid working and playing outside whenever possible during the month or season that bothers you the most. Stay inside when pollen counts are highest, which is in the morning or early evening or on dry, windy days. Peak pollen times are usually between 10 A.M. and 4 P.M. If you have to go outside, wear a face mask that filters out pollen and prevents it from getting into your nose.

▸ Keep your bedroom windows closed during allergy season to prevent any pollen from getting in. If you have to close your

A normal peak flow rate varies from person to person. Your doctor will help you determine what is normal for you. Once you have determined it, you can recognize changes or trends in your rate.

Encourage your doctor to establish an *asthma action plan* to guide you in the ongoing treatment of your asthma. When you measure your peak flow, it will fall in one of three zones—green, yellow, or red. Green means you are at 80 to 100 percent of your normal peak flow rate, and everything is fine. Yellow means you are at 50 to 80 percent of your normal peak flow rate and you should take caution—your airways are narrowing and you may require treatment. You and your doctor should discuss how to handle yellow readings so you are prepared in the event that you get one. If your reading is less than 50 percent of your normal, you are in the red zone. Your airways are severely narrowed, and you need to take your rescue medication right away.

Measure your peak flow rate at around the same times every day. Your doctor can help you determine the best times, but a common suggestion is to measure it twice a day—between 7 and 9 A.M. and between 6 and 8 P.M. You or a parent or guardian can obtain a peak flow meter at most pharmacies or from pharmaceutical companies, and many doctors give them out for free.

windows during a hot time of the year, make sure you have an air conditioner to prevent your room from getting too stuffy. Don't use window fans—they draw in air from the outside and, therefore, pollen.

▶ Shower, wash your hair, and put on fresh clothing as soon as you come in from outside to rid yourself of any pollen that you may have carried in.

▶ During the time of year when your pollen allergies are flaring, keep car windows closed whenever you drive or ride in a car.

▶ Make sure your house is not surrounded by weeds. Pull weeds or use a weed killer to get rid of them (but make sure someone other than you pulls them out). Stay away from zinnias, mums, dahlias, and sunflowers. They may be pretty, but they are relatives of ragweed—one of the biggest causes of pollen allergies.

‣ Before you head out, check the pollen forecast in your area by calling your local weather network, by looking at an online weather site, or by calling the National Allergy Bureau at 1-800-9POLLEN.

‣ Talk to your parents about planning a family vacation to a pollen-free place such as the beach—at the time of year when your pollen allergies are the worst—to give you a break.

MOLD ALLERGY

Like pollen, mold can be tricky to avoid because it grows pretty much everywhere there is moisture. Molds are fungi that thrive on decaying plant life and give off spores that can be inhaled, but you can reduce your exposure by doing the following:

‣ Whenever possible, steer clear of "moldy" places, such as moist, shady areas, damp basements and closets, bathrooms (this is tough, but you can keep your time spent in the bathroom to a minimum), greenhouses, mills, grain fields, garbage pails, moldy mattresses, upholstered furniture, and old foam rubber pillows.

‣ After you take a steamy shower, open a window in the bathroom or turn on an exhaust fan to remove the moisture.

‣ Before you spend time in a potentially moldy indoor space, such as a summer cabin or beach house, make sure it has been aired out sufficiently.

‣ Be sure that your yard is mowed and raked regularly to keep mold from growing. Ideally, a family member should do the mowing or raking. If you have to do it, wear a tightly fitting dust mask to protect your nose from the mold spores.

‣ During the time of year when crops are being harvested, avoid traveling to the country or walking through tall vegetation.

‣ Avoid tile floors or walls in bathrooms—the grouting encourages mold growth and is hard to keep clean.

‣ Remove all plants from inside the house, or cover the soil with aluminum foil to prevent moisture from the soil from getting into the air. There are also substances you can add to potting soil to prevent mold growth.

‣ Make sure all rooms in your house are well dusted, especially your bedroom.

➤ Use a dehumidifier to take the moisture out of your basement and other damp rooms, and make sure the machine is cleaned up regularly to avoid mold growth there. Aim for between 40 and 50 percent humidity in your home.

➤ Make sure the rain spouts on the side of your house aren't directing rainwater too close to the foundation, and make sure all drains are working properly.

➤ Clean air conditioners, furnace filters, vaporizers, humidifiers, and dehumidifiers regularly to prevent the growth of mold.

➤ Get rid of old furniture, rags, and carpeting—they are a haven for mold growth.

➤ Ideally, to avoid dampness, recreation areas in your home should not be built below ground level. Best-case scenario: There is no basement or cellar.

➤ If there is a mudroom in your house, it should be separate from the living areas, so damp and muddy shoes, boots, and sneakers can dry out by themselves.

➤ Install a dehumidifier in damp rooms in your house, such as the basement.

➤ If you have an unfinished basement, the walls should be painted with mold-resistant paint.

➤ Be sure that your dryer is properly ventilated so it pumps moisture to the outdoors.

➤ Clean shower curtains, shower walls, bathroom windowsills, damp walls, areas with dry rot, and indoor trash cans with a mixture of 50 percent water, 50 percent chlorine bleach, at least once a month.

➤ Use an electric fan to ventilate rooms with few windows.

➤ Make sure all crawl spaces in your house have adequate drainage to get rid of standing water. Cover the crawl space floor with polyethylene sheets to reduce dampness even more.

➤ Keep up to date on the latest environmental control measures. *Consumer Reports* rates these products now and then, and new ones are constantly coming out.

PET ALLERGY

If you are allergic to your dog or cat, the fastest and most effective way to get rid of your allergies is to get rid of the animal. Even if you do, it may take up to six months for all traces of your pet—and therefore your allergies—to disappear. Getting rid of a pet is not an easy solution, however, because you and your family members have probably grown attached to Spot or Whiskers. If you cannot bear to see your pet(s) go, here are some things you can do to ease the sniffling and sneezing you experience in their presence:

- Remove all carpeting and soft furnishings that have trapped animal dander and dried proteins from your pets' saliva and skin.
- Treat your animal with special shampoos and chemical products that help make their dander less allergenic. One product is called Allerpet. Your vet or pet store can recommend other treatment products. If you have a cat, have a friend or family member bathe it weekly and brush it outdoors every few days.
- Wear a face mask whenever you clean. Use vacuum cleaners and room cleaners that contain *HEPA filters.*
- As nice as it is to fall asleep next to your furry friend, keep your pet out of your bedroom at all times.
- Keep the pet(s) outside of the house as often as possible.
- When the pet dies, don't assume you will be safe if you choose a different animal. People with pet allergies are often allergic to numerous different animals.
- Ask babysitters and other visitors to wear clothes that have not been exposed to their pets if they have animals.
- In addition to live animals, stay away from clothing made of cashmere, goat hair, alpaca, and mohair, as well as horsehair-stuffed chairs and couches and feather and down pillows. Instead, stick to things made from synthetic materials.
- If you know you are going to visit a friend or relative who has a pet, take an antihistamine or your asthma medication *before* you leave so you will be able to better tolerate the animal. If you are planning to stay overnight, make sure the pet doesn't sleep in the same room with you and that the room and bedding have been thoroughly cleaned.

FOOD ALLERGY

Many people think they are allergic to foods, but few of them have food allergies in their true form. What they actually have are food sensitivities. People with bona fide food allergies have a potentially dangerous situation on their hands, and they need to avoid the food(s) in question in order to prevent a dangerous anaphylactic reaction. The top 10 foods that are responsible for food allergies are peanuts (which is not a nut but a legume), tree nuts (e.g., walnuts, almonds), fish, shellfish, eggs, milk, soy, wheat, and sesame seeds. Beyond avoiding the food you are allergic to like the plague, here are some things you can do if you have a food allergy:

- ▸ Read food labels very carefully to check for your trigger food. Since January 2006, all food manufacturers are required to list whether a food contains one of the most common food allergens. Sometimes foods are listed as ingredients in products you would never suspect. For example, peanut oil is often used in Asian cooking, and eggs can be found in cookies and pastries.
- ▸ Ask your health care professional for a list of the various names of different forms of the food you should avoid. Peanuts, for example, can be hidden in a number of ingredients, and you must be familiar with all of them in order to totally avoid the nut.
- ▸ If you are extremely sensitive to a food, even touching it may give you a reaction. Make sure you wash your hands each time there is a chance you could have been exposed to the food you are sensitive to, as well as before you eat.
- ▸ When you eat at a restaurant, make sure you ask about the ingredients in any dish you order to make sure it doesn't contain the food to which you are allergic.
- ▸ Do not share utensils and be careful of *cross-contamination,* where a utensil may have touched a food allergen and then been used to prepare your meal.
- ▸ If you have a severe food allergy, be sure to wear a *Medic Alert bracelet or necklace* and carry a syringe containing epinephrine (EpiPen or Twinject) at all times. You can get a prescription for the injection from your doctor.
- ▸ Avoid close contact to a person who has recently eaten the substance to which you are allergic. Kissing someone who has recently consumed something like peanut butter may be very dangerous if you are allergic to peanuts.

INSECT BITE OR STING ALLERGY

More than 2 million Americans are allergic to insect bites or stings, and 50 to 150 deaths and up to 1 million hospital visits occur each year as a result of them. The majority of insects that cause the potentially life-threatening anaphylactic reaction are bees, yellow jackets, hornets, wasps, and fire ants. In addition to avoiding these insects if you see them, here are some things you can do to avoid being bitten or stung:

▸ Avoid wearing loose-fitting clothing, which can trap insects. Instead, wear clothing that covers your arms and legs when you go outside.

▸ If a bee or wasp lands on you, do not slap it or make jerking movements. Instead, gently blow it away. If a bee flies into your car, do not panic. Roll down all the windows, and it will probably fly out.

▸ Wear the right colors. White, green, tan, and khaki are attractive to insects, as are bright colors and floral patterns and materials like denim and corduroy. So to avoid insects, steer clear of these materials and shades.

▸ Be careful around birdbaths, pet bowls, and puddles—insects like to feed in these moist places.

▸ Refrain from wearing colognes, perfumes, hair sprays, or scented lotions when you go outside.

▸ Steer clear of clover bushes, shrubs, large rocks, logs, woodpiles, eaves of buildings, and shutters—they all harbor insect nests.

▸ Keep picnic food covered and approach areas with food carefully.

▸ In the event that you are stung, try to remove the stinger to avoid getting more venom into your skin. Use a knife edge or fingernail to gently flick the stinger out of your skin—do not pinch it.

DEVICES THAT HELP EASE ALLERGY SYMPTOMS

Teens who suffer from allergies today are much better off than those who suffered centuries ago. These days, there are a range of household devices that can help reduce your exposure to the allergens that bother you. In addition to the other measures mentioned throughout this chapter, here are some of the available devices that can help cut down on allergens in your environment:

Dehumidifier. To keep mold growth and dust mites under control, you (or your parents) may want to invest in a dehumidifier. With all the showering, cooking, and laundry that goes on in the typical family home, humidity is a common problem. To avoid excess mold and mites, keep the humidity level between 40 and 50 percent relative humidity. (Humidity is the amount of moisture in the air; relative humidity is the percentage of the maximum amount of moisture the air can hold at a given temperature). A dehumidifier will help keep the moisture level in your home constant and under control. It works by drawing indoor air over cooling coils, which condenses the moisture into water droplets that fall into a bucket or floor drain.

Special vacuum cleaner. Although standard vacuum cleaners do a great job of picking up house dust and other particles, for the dust allergy sufferer, they can make things worse because they blow out some dust as they clean. A central vacuum with an outside vent in the basement will prevent dust from being recirculated. Easy Flo is a central vacuum cleaner recommended by *Consumer Reports.* If your family would rather not invest in a central vacuum, you can also use a standard vacuum cleaner with a HEPA filter system, such as Oreck.

Air filters. An air filter is a mechanical filter that physically traps particles in the air. Charcoal filters absorb particles and odors like cooking fumes and cigarette smoke, and electronic filters remove bigger particles from the air. Most respiratory organizations and physicians recommend HEPA filters as the most effective type. (HEPA stands for high efficiency particulate arresting.) One study that compared HEPA filters to blank air filters in patients' homes found that the patients with the HEPA filters had fewer symptoms and required less medication than those with the blank filters. Small air filters work best when they are installed in your bedroom. To find the best air filter for your needs, consult your physician. If he or she recommends a HEPA filter, your parents may be able to obtain a tax refund for their purchase of one.

Furnace filter. Another air purification option is a furnace filter. Installed in your furnace, these filters work similarly to the way electrostatic charges pick up small pieces of paper in that they are made of materials that are positively and negatively charged. When air goes through the filter, pollen and dust are zapped before they have a chance to circulate in the air you breathe. Furnace filters are inexpensive (they cost $100 to $300), they are easy to install, they require little maintenance (they have to be washed every two months), and they remain effective long-term.

Air conditioner. When it comes to preventing allergy symptoms, air conditioners work in two ways. For one, they help remove particles like mold spores, dust, and pollen from the air. And second, they help keep pollen and other outdoor allergens from getting in the house by keeping the house cool with the windows closed. For maximum effectiveness, air conditioner coils and filters should be cleaned regularly, and the temperature controls shouldn't be set too low—air that is too cold can worsen breathing problems.

OVERALL ALLERGY-PROOFING TIPS

In addition to the actions discussed above, there are some things you and/or your family members can do to make your house more resistant to allergens, no matter what it is you are allergic to:

▸ If possible, avoid heating the house with a blower furnace; use electric or hot water heat instead.
▸ Make sure all appliances, including refrigerators, TVs, radios, DVD players, and dishwashers, can be moved in order to clean the dust, food particles, and insects that hide out underneath them.
▸ Be sure that doors and windows fit tightly and have screens to keep outdoor pollutants out.
▸ Keep knickknacks to a minimum—not only do they attract dust but they create safe spots for insects to breed.
▸ Paint cement floors and basement walls with special paints that are waterproof, inhibit dust formation, and prevent mold growth.
▸ Put the washing machine and dryer in a room that is vented to the outside.
▸ Avoid having a lot of shrubbery around the house. Trim trees, brushes, and hedges regularly.
▸ Place garbage cans and receptacles in a shed to protect them from animals and birds.

IDENTIFYING EARLY SIGNS OF AN ATTACK

Even with the most sterile environment, there is sometimes nothing you can do to prevent an allergy attack, and you cannot always stay in areas that are allergen-free. So in addition to doing all that is in your power to control your own space, you should be prepared to act in the event that a serious attack strikes while you are away.

The most life-threatening allergy attack is anaphylaxis, sometimes referred to as anaphylactic shock, and usually results from exposure to a food allergen, medication such as antibiotics, or insect sting, and it may involve the entire body. Symptoms of anaphylaxis may begin in as little as one to 15 minutes of exposure to the allergen, but a life-threatening reaction may progress over several hours. Symptoms include:

- Skin: Hives, swelling, flushing of the face or body, tingling or warm sensation
- Gastrointestinal: Stomach cramping, vomiting, diarrhea, difficulty swallowing
- Circulatory system: Severe drop in blood pressure
- Respiratory system: Chest tightness, throat tightness, wheezing, coughing, difficulty breathing
- Mental: Loss of consciousness, feeling faint, sense of fear
- Taste: A metallic taste in the mouth

To ensure that you and the people around you know what to do in the event of an allergy emergency, there are a few actions you can take. First, make sure you wear a Medic Alert bracelet or necklace. Medic Alert devices are engraved with your medical condition, membership number, and the 24-hour emergency response number (1-888-904-7629). Paramedics are trained to look for Medic Alert devices right away so they can act appropriately. Also, carry an epinephrine injection kit such as EpiPen or Twinject wherever you go.

BE PREPARED: DEVELOP AN ALLERGY ACTION AND TREATMENT PLAN

If you suffer from allergies, an allergy action and treatment plan is a great tool for you to have. First, it will help you better understand the nature of your allergies and what you can do when they strike. Second, it will give you peace of mind to know you are prepared in the event of a surprise attack. To help you develop your action and treatment plan, the Asthma and Allergy Foundation of America has created an easy-to-use screening tool that you can access online at http://www.allergyactionplan.com/tool.html. In addition, the following resources—the allergy action plan and allergy emergency plan—will help you and others around you recognize allergy symptoms, provide information on prescription and over-the-counter medications, and give special instructions for special circumstances and potential emergencies. If you have allergies, particularly if they may be life threatening, you should carry all three plans with you at all times so your friends, teachers, and coaches all know what to do should you suffer an attack. It is a good idea to include a copy of the instructions for your Twinject or EpiPen along with each of your action plans.

ALLERGY ACTION PLAN

Name: _____

Grade: _____ Date of birth: _____

Name of parent or guardian: _____

Phone numbers:

(H)_____ (W)_____

Address:_____

Other contact info: _____

Emergency phone contact #1

Name:_____ Relationship: _____

Phone: (H) _____ (W) _____

Emergency phone contact #2

Name: _____ Relationship: _____

Phone: (H) _____ (W) _____

Physician teen sees for asthma/allergies: _____

Phone: _____

Other physician: _____

Phone: _____

Medications and/or dietary restrictions necessary to prevent an allergy/asthma episode:_____

Comments:_____

Peak flow monitoring (for children under four years old) _____

Personal best peak flow reading: _____

Monitoring times:_____

Check the things that start an allergy/asthma episode:

☐ Animals   ☐ Chalk dust

☐ Bee/insect stings   ☐ Latex

☐ Dust mites   ☐ Change in temperature

☐ Pollens   ☐ Strong odors

☐ Molds   ☐ Respiratory infections

☐ Food; list types: _____

Daily medication plan for allergies/asthma:

Name:_____ Amount: _____

When to use:_____

Outside activities and field trips:
The following medications must accompany the child during any
outside activities or field trips:

Name: _____ Amount: _____

When to use: _____

ALLERGY EMERGENCY PLAN

Child's name:_____

Date of birth: _____

Teacher: _____

Child is allergic to: _____

Asthmatic?   yes   no

Emergency action is necessary when the child has the following symptoms: _____

Steps to take in the event of an allergy attack:

1. If any of the following symptoms occur, give the medications listed on the allergy action plan: shortness of breath, wheezing, coughing, nausea, abdominal cramps, vomiting, diarrhea, weak pulse, fainting, asthma symptoms.

2. Contact emergency help and ask for epinephrine.

3. Contact the parent or guardian.

4. Seek emergency medical care if the child has any of the following symptoms (allergy sufferer should work with physician to circle all that apply):

   ☐ No improvement is observed after first treatment with medications.

   ☐ Peak flow at or below _____ .

   ☐ Mouth, lips, or throat are swollen, itchy, or tight, or there is hoarseness or a cough.

   ☐ Child is having a hard time breathing.

   ☐ There are hives or there is a swollen or itchy rash.

   ☐ Child is hunched over.

   ☐ Child is having trouble walking or talking.

   ☐ Lips and/or fingernails are blue or gray.

(Together with your physician, circle the medication that should be given for each of the symptoms described below). It is good idea to include a copy of the instructions for Twinject or EpiPen along with your actions plans.

   ▶ It a food allergen has been ingested but there are no symptoms:

   ☐ Twinject or EpiPen

   ☐ Antihistamine

   ☐ Other: _____

➤ Shortness or breath, wheezing, repetitive coughing

 ☐ Twinject or EpiPen

 ☐ Antihistamine

 ☐ Other: _____

➤ Swelling, tingling or itching of the mouth, tongue, or lips

 ☐ Twinject or EpiPen

 ☐ Antihistamine

 ☐ Other: _____

➤ Nausea, abdominal cramps, vomiting, diarrhea

 ☐ Twinject or EpiPen

 ☐ Antihistamine

 ☐ Other: _____

➤ Tightening of the throat, cough, hoarse voice

 ☐ Twinject or EpiPen

 ☐ Antihistamine

 ☐ Other: _____

➤ Hives, itchy rash, swelling or the extremities or face

 ☐ Twinject or EpiPen

 ☐ Antihistamine

 ☐ Other: _____

➤ Weak pulse, low blood pressure, pale or blue color, fainting

 ☐ Twinject or EpiPen

 ☐ Antihistamine

 ☐ Other: _____

Special instructions: _____

_____

Emergency contacts:

   1. name:_____   relationship: _____

      phone numbers:_____

   2. name:_____   relationship: _____

      phone numbers: _____

   3. name:_____   relationship: _____

      phone numbers:_____

   4. name:_____   relationship: _____

      phone numbers:_____

Even if parent/guardian or emergency contacts cannot be reached, do not hesitate to medicate or call 911.

Parent/guardian signature:_____

Date: _____

Physician signature (required): _____

Date: _____

Here are some guidelines to help you decide when to call the doctor and when to seek emergency medical help for allergies or asthma. For allergies, emergency medical help is necessary when a patient experiences any symptoms of anaphylactic shock:

- *Skin*: Hives, swelling, flushing of the face or body, tingling or warm sensation
- *Gastrointestinal*: Stomach cramping, vomiting, diarrhea, difficulty swallowing
- *Respiratory*: Chest tightness, throat tightness, wheezing, coughing, difficulty breathing
- *Circulatory*: Drop in blood pressure with resultant dizziness or loss of consciousness
- *Taste*: A metallic taste in the mouth

In most other cases, a call to the doctor to ask for advice is sufficient. You should, however, discuss with your doctor the specific symptoms that indicate you should seek emergency medical help. Everyone is different, and he or she may want you to act more quickly than some people in the event that you are exposed to a certain allergen.

For asthma, you should seek emergency medical help and call 911 if:

▸ You are having severe difficulty breathing.
▸ You feel like you are going to pass out.
▸ Wheezing started suddenly after you ate a food, were stung by an insect, or took a certain medication.

Call your doctor right away if:

▸ You feel very sick.
▸ You look like you did when you were hospitalized with asthma before.
▸ You are having trouble breathing, and it does not subside 20 minutes after using an inhaler.
▸ Your peak flow rate is lower than 50 percent of normal.
▸ Your peak flow rate is 50 to 80 percent of normal after you used an inhaler.
▸ Wheezing doesn't go away 20 minutes after using an inhaler.
▸ You have nonstop coughing that keeps you from playing or sleeping.
▸ You need your asthma medicine more frequently than every four hours.
▸ You have a fever higher than 104 degrees Fahrenheit.
▸ You have severe chest pain.

Call your doctor within 24 hours (during business hours) if:

▸ You think you need to be seen.
▸ You have sinus pressure or pain.
▸ Your have a fever that lasts more than three days.

WHAT YOU NEED TO KNOW

▸ When it comes to allergies, prevention is often the best treatment.
▸ Your family should avoid using insect sprays or pesticide bombs to get rid of cockroaches—they can cause asthma symptoms worse than those caused by the cockroaches themselves.
▸ Before you head out, check the pollen forecast in your area by calling your local weather network, by looking at an online

weather site, or by calling the National Allergy Bureau at 1-800-9POLLEN.

➤ Keep up to date on the latest environmental control measures to help keep your allergies under control. *Consumer Reports* rates these products now and then, and new ones are constantly coming out.

➤ If you are allergic to your dog or cat, the fastest and most effective way to get rid of your allergies is to get rid of the animal. Even if you do, it may take up to six months for all traces of your pet—and therefore your allergies—to disappear.

➤ Many people think they are allergic to foods, but few of them have food allergies in their true form. What they actually have are food sensitivities. People with bonafide food allergies have a potentially dangerous situation on their hands, and they need to avoid the food(s) in question in order to prevent a dangerous anaphylactic reaction.

➤ If you have a severe food allergy or an allergy to insect bites or stings, be sure to wear a Medic Alert bracelet or necklace and carry a syringe containing epinephrine (EpiPen or Twinject) at all times. You can get a prescription for the injection from your doctor.

➤ To help you develop your action and treatment plan, the Asthma and Allergy Foundation of America has created an easy-to-use screening tool that you can access online at http://www.allergyactionplan.com/tool.html.

6

Allergies at School

As a teen with allergies, your backpack will be filled with more than pencils and notebooks on the first day of school; you will probably also need to remember your medications. You probably already know that keeping your allergies under control at school is more difficult than controlling them at home. In your own house, you always know your medications—and your mom or dad—are just a few feet away. You also know that the environment is controlled to help prevent your allergies from flaring up. When you get to school, however, things are a little different. You no longer have the security of being in your own house, and the threat of being exposed to the thing you are allergic to looms large. This is particularly true if you have a potentially life-threatening food allergy. However, if your teachers, coaches, and peers are well educated about your allergies and what they entail, they will be equally as prepared to recognize and help you treat an attack as your parents.

Another reason allergies present a different kind of problem at school is that classrooms can be a breeding ground for allergens. If a school is poorly ventilated and damp (which many are), allergy-causing mold will grow there. Guinea pigs and white mice add a nice educational component to science classes, but they are also full of allergens. The beginning-of-school time of year also leads to air temperature inversions (when warm air sits on top of cold) both indoors and outdoors, which leads to a buildup of contaminants. Then, when heating season starts, all the dust and mouse droppings that were sitting in the furnace all summer and fall get

73

blown through the heating ducts and into the classrooms. Also, all through the year, chalk, pollens, pests, pesticides, sanitation supplies, laboratory chemicals, rodents, perfumes, and cockroaches in schools pose a threat seven to 10 hours a day. So it's no surprise that students with certain allergies start to sniffle and sneeze. No matter what your allergy, to avoid it at school, the best thing you can do as you start a new school year is have an allergy treatment plan in place *before* the first day.

YOUR BACK-TO-SCHOOL PLAN

As you prepare for a new school year with clothes shopping and catching up with friends, you may find it hard to concentrate on developing an at-school allergy or asthma treatment plan. In high school, you may be more concerned with friendships, sports, dating, and picking classes than you are with carrying your EpiPen or inhaler, but you must remember that unless your allergies or asthma are well-controlled, these conditions will interfere with your ability to get the most out of your high school years. That's why a clear, easy-to-follow school allergy action and/or emergency plan is vitally important, both for you and the people who will surround you at school.

One thing to keep in mind is that you are not alone. Thousands of teens in private and public schools across the country deal with allergies and asthma every day, and there are probably more than a few in your very own school. According to the Environmental Protection Agency, asthma accounts for more than 10 million missed school days per year. In fact, asthma is the leading cause of school absenteeism from a chronic illness.

Overall, remember that *you* are your best first line of defense. You have the power to protect yourself by carrying your medications at all times and by doing what you can to make sure your environment is as allergen-free as possible. Before your first day, set up a meeting between you, a parent, your homeroom teacher, school nurse, cafeteria staff, and school principal. At the meeting, discuss your allergies or asthma, which medications you need and when, and any special instructions, such as dietary limitations or avoiding certain substances. Also ask your school administrator if there is a policy for what needs to be done before you can carry and take your medications. For example, some schools require a signed form from your doctor; in New York City, students are not permitted to bring any medication to school—even aspirin—without a signed Form 504.

CARRYING YOUR MEDICATION

When it comes to carrying your allergy medications at school, luckily, the law is on your side. Under civil rights law 504, children and teenagers with allergies cannot be discriminated against and must be accommodated during the school day. The law says that if your classrooms are near the nurse's office and the nurse is there at all times to administer the drug you need, then it can be kept in there with him or her. If you do not have immediate access to the nurse's office (which is usually the case in middle and high school), you need a plan that will permit you to carry your medicines with you at all times.

If you need to carry epinephrine (EpiPen or Twinject) because you have a life-threatening allergy to food or insect stings, you are legally permitted to carry the medication in your purse, pocket, or backpack. The American Academy of Allergy, Asthma & Immunology (AAAAI) policy on school administration of epinephrine says that older responsible children and teenagers may carry epinephrine on them, and teachers and others should be trained to administer the drug in the event that you cannot do it yourself. (It is a good idea to keep a copy of the instructions for Twinject or EpiPen in your purse or backpack—along with your action plans—so those around you have clear instructions on what to do in an emergency.)

If you need an asthma inhaler, your school administrator will probably let you carry it with you during the day if you have a note from your doctor. As a teen with asthma, you have the right to have access to your rescue medication at all times.

Carrying an action plan and your medications with you does not make you exempt from taking care regarding your allergies, however. You may feel that since you are armed with an EpiPen or an inhaler, you can partake in the same freedoms as your friends. Unfortunately, this is not the case. Although a good action plan and a constant dose of medication (just in case) will keep you more protected in the event of an attack, it is still your responsibility to avoid certain high-risk situations. For example, if you have a peanut allergy, you simply cannot sit at a crowded table filled with people who are unaware of the danger that nuts pose to you. Or if you have an allergy to insect stings, you have to be more mindful about being near food outside, or about playing sports in areas where there may be stinging insects' nests. The more you take chances, the more things can go wrong. Just as the percentages are against teenagers when they drive, they are against you when you push the limits of your allergy medication regimen.

State and City Laws Regarding Teens Carrying Medication

The laws governing teens carrying medications vary from state to state. To find out the laws that apply to the state you live in, go to http://www.schoolasthmaallergy.com/html/states/index.html.

Because most middle and high school students change classes regularly, it's also a good idea for you to have multiple EpiPens or Twinjects at school. Put one in your backpack, purse, or the bag that you carry with you throughout the day. If you don't carry a bag, make sure you have an EpiPen or Twinject in your pocket. Cargo pants are a good option for boys who do not want to carry a bag. As a backup, keep one in your locker, and if your teachers agree—which they definitely should—ask each one of them to keep an EpiPen or Twinject in their desks as well, so you, they, or a classmate can get to it quickly in the event that you have an attack. If you ride the bus, also give one to your bus driver.

In addition to your teachers and bus driver, if it is severe, make sure all your friends and classmates are aware of your allergy. There is nothing to be embarrassed about; plenty of teenagers have allergies, and your classmates will probably be happy that you informed them, so they can help in the event of an attack.

During an allergy attack at school, always err on the side of caution. If you are able, give yourself an epinephrine (EpiPen or Twinject) shot the moment you start to experience symptoms. The only known side effect of epinephrine is a racing heart, so it can't hurt you to take it, even if it turns out that it wasn't necessary. Make sure you tell your friends the same thing—if they see you suffering in any way, they should give you the shot, no questions asked.

DEALING WITH DIFFERENT TYPES OF ALLERGIES AT SCHOOL

Different allergies require different actions. Here is an overview of common allergies and how they should be dealt with at school:

Allergic rhinitis. If you have nasal allergies, you may not require a school action plan to treat them, unless they are severe. You should do your best to avoid indoor allergens that trigger your allergies, such as dust, classroom animals, chalk dust, and mold. In most cases, you can probably just take your allergy medication in the morning, before you leave for school. If you experience a lot of symptoms at school and you think you should take your medication during the day, check with your doctor.

Food allergies. Food allergies are fairly common in school-aged children; six to eight percent of students have a food allergy, half of which have a high risk of life-threatening anaphylaxis. Peanuts and tree nuts make up 92 percent of potentially fatal reactions, but other foods such as shellfish, soy, fish, and even mustard can also cause severe attacks. If you have a food allergy, it is imperative that you have a thorough school emergency plan in case you accidentally ingest or are exposed to the food to which you are allergic. (See the sidebar with emergency action plan on page 82.) You can give this plan to every school official you encounter throughout the day. Also, before the start of the school year, sit down with your teachers, school nurse, and cafeteria staff to help ensure that you completely avoid your trigger food. Your risk of accidental ingestion will go down considerably if you involve both your physician and your school administrators in the process.

It is also very important that you have injectable epinephrine (EpiPen or Twinject) available at school at all times to treat a severe food allergy if you accidentally ingest the food. You should carry a dose in your purse, backpack, or in your pocket; and for maximum safety, all your teachers, the nurse, and the cafeteria staff should have one on hand as well—plus a copy of your allergy emergency plan—so you can be treated as quickly as possible.

In addition to doing everything you can to avoid your trigger food, you should follow the following rules:

▸ Do not trade food with classmates.
▸ Do not eat anything that is known to contain your allergen or contains unknown ingredients.
▸ Notify an adult immediately if you think you ate something that contains the food to which you are allergic.
▸ If you have a food allergy, you may want to sit at a designated "peanut-free" or "shellfish-free" table to minimize your chances of exposure.
▸ Be proactive in the care and management of your food allergy.

For further information, the Food Allergy and Anaphylaxis Network (http://www.foodallergy.org) offers guidance on food allergies and is a valuable resource to help you deal with your food allergies, both in and out of school.

Venom and stinging insect allergy. Bees and other stinging insects can be difficult to avoid at school. They buzz around school campuses, especially at times when there is food outside, such as during sporting events or picnics. When the weather is warm, they often fly into open windows and throughout classrooms. If you are allergic

Riding the School Bus with Allergies

As a middle or high school student, you may or may not take the bus to school. If you do, you need to arm your bus driver with the same tools to deal with an allergy attack as you've given to teachers and administrators at school. Here are some steps you or your parents can take:

▶ Make sure that your bus driver is armed with a cell phone and knows to call 911 in the event that you suffer an attack while riding to and from school.

▶ Include the bus driver in the same training that the school nurse and other school administrators had regarding how to treat your allergy.

▶ Consider sitting in the front of the bus, near the driver.

▶ Ensure that your bus driver has enforced a "no food on the bus" rule.

▶ Carry an EpiPen or Twinject in your purse or backpack at all times while riding the bus and give the driver a copy of your emergency action plan.

▶ If you are not comfortable riding the bus, consider driving yourself to school (if you have a license), getting a ride from a parent or guardian, or riding with friends who understand the severity of your allergy and know what to do in an emergency.

to insect stings, it is important that you carry injectable epinephrine with you at all times in case you are stung. That way, you can quickly give yourself a shot—or hand the EpiPen or Twinject to a friend to give the shot to you—if you are having an attack. As a backup, you should give an injection kit and a copy of your allergy emergency plan to your school nurse and one or all of your teachers as well.

WHEN SYMPTOMS OCCUR *ONLY* AT SCHOOL

On days when you didn't want to get out of bed, you may have been tempted to tell your mom or dad that you are allergic to school, but if your allergy symptoms pop up soon—and only—after you set foot in your school building, an allergy to school may not be so far-fetched. If this is the case, you can start by thinking like a detective. When you experience symptoms, look around you. Is there chalk dust? A pet or animal in the classroom? New carpeting or dust from building construction? Or does your teacher use air fresheners, wear colognes or perfumes, or other artificial scents? If so, any one of these factors could be causing your symptoms. Make sure you consider the things you are exposed to at school outside the classroom as well, such as the trees and pollens on sports fields or the weeds growing outside open classroom windows.

Beyond the detective work, if you suspect you are allergic to something in your environment at school, first, if you haven't already, visit an allergist, immunologist, or your family doctor and explain your symptoms. They can advise you on the appropriate ways to prevent symptoms, and they can prescribe medication or immunotherapy, if necessary. You can also take a tour of the school with your parent and an administrator to look for potential allergens, such as classroom pets, dust, and mold. Also, don't be afraid to talk to your teachers about what they can do to help. If you tell them about the symptoms you are having, they may work with you to develop a more allergy-free environment in their classrooms. Once you or your parents have talked to your teachers about your symptoms, here is a checklist you can give to them to help minimize the allergic classroom environments:

▸ Make sure classrooms are cleaned regularly so dust does not accumulate.
▸ During high pollen seasons, keep windows closed whenever possible.
▸ If you have a chemically sensitive student in your classroom, consider projects that don't involve known irritants.

> If you use a chalkboard, assign allergic students seats in the back of the classroom.
> If you have students who are allergic to animals, choose your classroom pets carefully. Instead of animals with fur, consider a reptile or an aquarium.
> Make sure cleaning with harsh chemical solutions is done after hours or at night, when there are no students in the building.
> Consider talking with the school administrator about putting an air purifier in the classroom—everyone will breathe easier.

ASTHMA AT SCHOOL

If you are a teen with asthma, you know that the disruption of routines, sleeplessness, and activity limitations associated with asthma all take a toll on your ability to concentrate in class and do homework, as well as on your general quality of life. Asthma is most likely to flare up at times of exercise, such as during sports practice or in gym class, when you are exposed to allergens in or outside of the classroom, or when you are sick. In classrooms with chalkboards, you may notice that your asthma symptoms are worse. If this is the case, ask the teacher if you can sit in the back of the room, away from the chalkboard, avoid the chalkboard erasers (a nice excuse to get out of erasing the board!), and wash your hands after you handle chalk.

Outside at school, cold air, exercise, or outdoor dust or mold exposure can cause asthma to flare up. To prevent it, your doctor may recommend you use your rescue medication or inhaler before you have gym class or you know you will be exercising strenuously outside.

If you have a serious allergy that is either food-related or exercise-induced, your gym teacher should be properly trained to recognize your symptoms and trained to respond appropriately if you suffer an attack. In addition, if you must remove a medical alert bracelet for gym class, be mindful to put it back on immediately after class is over.

GOING ON SCHOOL FIELD TRIPS WITH ALLERGIES OR ASTHMA

As a student, field trips can be some of the greatest experiences you have in middle or high school. Not only do you get to take a break from sitting in class but you have the opportunity to visit an interesting place and learn something new. Field trips can be some of the most effective learning experiences you have in grade school. So as a student with allergies or asthma, you certainly shouldn't be excluded from these fun and educational trips. If your allergy is life-threatening, your teachers will have to choose field trips for your class that put you at the lowest possible risk of an attack. If you have a peanut allergy, a peanut farm or a peanut butter factory, for example, are definitely out of the question. Your school nurse will probably be the one responsible for determining the appropriateness of each field trip.

Whenever you travel on field trips, you will have to do some preparation. You and the chaperone should carry a copy of your allergy action plan and/or emergency plan, which should include the name and phone number of the nearest hospital. If your allergy is life-threatening, the school nurse may accompany you on the trip. If he or she cannot make it, a parent, registered nurse, or another individual specifically trained to watch out for your welfare and act in the case of an emergency, should come with you. Any meals you eat on field trips should be packaged carefully to avoid cross-contamination with other students' meals, and you should clean your hands with hand wipes before and after you eat. Needless to say, if you are not packing your own meal, any meal that could contain your allergen should be avoided.

WHAT *OTHERS* NEED TO KNOW: ALLERGY ACTION PLANS FOR SCHOOL

Together with your physician, you should develop a written allergy action plan specifically for school. Sample action plans appear in Chapter 5. Below is a sample food allergy action plan from the Food Allergy & Anaphylaxis Network. For children with multiple food allergies, consider providing separate action plans for different foods.

FOOD ALLERGY ACTION PLAN

(Place child's photo in the upper right hand corner)

Student's name: _____

D.O.B.: _____

Teacher: _____

Allergy to: _____

Asthmatic? Yes*_____ No_____
*Higher risk for severe reaction

STEP 1: TREATMENT

Symptoms:	Give circled medication (To be determined by physician authorizing treatment)	
If food allergen has been ingested, but no symptoms	Epinephrine	Antihistamine
Mouth—itching, tingling, or swelling of the lips, tongue, mouth	Epinephrine	Antihistamine
Skin—hives, itchy rash, swelling of the face or extremities	Epinephrine	Antihistamine
Gut—nausea, abdominal cramps, vomiting, diarrhea	Epinephrine	Antihistamine
Throat**—tingling of throat, hoarseness, hacking cough	Epinephrine	Antihistamine
Lung**—shortness of breath, repetitive coughing, wheezing	Epinephrine	Antihistamine
Heart**—weak or thready pulse, low blood pressure, fainting, pale, blueness	Epinephrine	Antihistamine
Other**	Epinephrine	Antihistamine
If reaction is progressing (several of the above areas affected), give:	Epinephrine	Antihistamine

**Indicates potentially life-threatening symptom. The severity of symptoms can quickly change.

DOSAGE:
Epinephrine: inject intramuscularly (circle one)

EpiPen   EpiPen Jr.   Twinject 0.3mg   Twinject 0.15mg
(see reverse side for instructions)

Antihistamine: give _____

Other: give _____

IMPORTANT: Asthma inhalers and/or antihistamines cannot be depended on to replace epinephrine in anaphylaxis.

STEP 2: EMERGENCY CALLS

1. Call 911 (or rescue squad: _____) State that an allergic reaction has been treated, and additional epinephrine may be needed.

2. Dr. Phone:_____

3. Parent Phone: _____

4. Emergency contacts:
   Name/Relationship: Phone number(s)

   a._____ 1) _____ 2) _____

   b._____ 1) _____ 2) _____

EVEN IF PARENT/GUARDIAN CANNOT BE REACHED, DO NOT HESITATE TO MEDICATE OR TAKE CHILD TO MEDICAL FACILITY:

Parent/guardian's signature _____ Date _____

Doctor's signature_____ Date _____
                            (required)

Trained Staff Members

1._____ Room_____

2._____ Room_____

3._____ Room_____

EpiPen and EpiPen Jr. Directions
 ▸ Pull off gray activation cap.

 ▸ Hold black tip near outer thigh (always apply to thigh).

 ▸ Swing and jab firmly into outer thigh until Auto-injector mechanism functions. Hold in place and count to 10. Remove the EpiPen unit and massage the injection area for 10 seconds.

Twinject 0.3 mg and Twinject 0.15 mg Directions

➤ Remove caps labeled "1" and "2."

➤ Place rounded tip against outer thigh, press down hard until needle penetrates. Hold for 10 seconds, then remove.

Second Dose Administration

If symptoms don't improve after 10 minutes, administer second dose:

➤ Unscrew rounded tip. Pull syringe from barrel by holding blue collar at needle base.

➤ Slide yellow collar off plunger.

➤ Put needle into thigh through skin, push plunger down all the way, and remove.

Once EpiPen or Twinject is used, call the rescue squad. Take the used unit with you to the Emergency Room. Plan to stay for observation at the Emergency Room for at least four hours.

Medication checklist adapted from the Authorization of Emergency Treatment form developed by the Mount Sinai School of Medicine. Used with permission.

THE ROLE OF YOUR PHYSICIAN

When it comes to dealing with allergies at school, your allergist, pediatrician, or family physician can be one of your greatest allies. Involving a physician in your allergy care at school will give your concerns more attention than they might get if you are working alone. Together with your physician, you should develop a written allergy action plan specifically for school and request that he or she get in touch with the principal, school nurse, and other appropriate school staff.

Here are two sample letters your physician can use to address your school: The first is addressed to your school nurse and/or classroom teachers. The second letter is for students with asthma, addressed to your physical education teacher. Both samples are from the American College of Allergy, Asthma & Immunology.

Sample Letter to School Nurse and/or Classroom Teachers

Date: _____

Dear School Nurse or Classroom Instructor:

_____(Name of Student_____ is under my care for asthma or allergies (choose one). All of us—physicians, parents, and school personnel—want to do everything possible to provide a normal learning experience for this student. The following information and instructions are provided so that we may work together to meet this goal.

- ▶ Permit the student to remain in regular physical education classes. We encourage patients with asthma to decide their activity level on a day-to-day basis. If you feel inappropriate choices are being made, please contact me so that we can all help the student maintain as normal an activity level as possible.
- ▶ If the student begins to miss a great deal of school because of asthma or allergies, urge the parents to notify me.
- ▶ If this student is not performing well in school, is drowsy, irritable, lethargic, lacks endurance, or has headaches or nausea, please have the parents notify me. These problems may be due to his/her medical condition or to side effects of asthma or allergy medication. Once we know the problems, changes can be made.
- ▶ If medications are required for use in school, they will be listed on a separate form. Please permit the student to self-medicate when authorized by me and the parent to have medication for acute treatment readily available at all times.

We welcome your help.

Sincerely,

_____   _____
(Physician's signature)   (Parent's signature)

_____   _____
Address   Address

_____   _____
City, State, Zip   City, State, Zip

_____   _____
Telephone   Telephone

Sample Letter to Physical Education Teacher

Date: _____

Dear Physical Education Instructor:

_____(Name of Student_____ is under my care for asthma. Because exercise is important for the child with asthma, both physically and psychologically, I am providing information and instruction concerning this child's participation in physical activities.

- He/she should be permitted to remain in regular PE classes and should be permitted to engage in regular physical activities most of the time. However, during asthma episodes (characterized by cough, wheeze, shortness of breath), activities may have to be temporarily curtailed.
- Each child with asthma has a different limit of tolerance to exercise. Please permit the youngster to set his/her own pace on a daily basis. In particular, children with asthma may have difficulty "running laps" and playing competitive soccer and basketball; please do not "force" the child, but let the student participate at his own level. Swimming is usually well-tolerated and an excellent activity for children with asthma.
- Warm-up exercises are often useful in warding off wheezing episodes.
- We do not wish the student with asthma to feel "different." Please do what is necessary toward accomplishing this end.
- If this student does not have some problems with "endurance" sports, please permit him/her to take the following medications* before participating to prevent symptoms:

    Medications: _____
- In case of breathing difficulty, talk to the child reassuringly and calmly; have the child take prescribed medication. If the treatment is ineffective or symptoms are severe, notify the school nurse or parent immediately or call 911 if appropriate. Medication(s)* for acute treatment must be readily available.

    Medications: _____

We welcome your help.

*The student's parent has been given a "school medication request" form to transmit to the school. Where indicated, permit the child to medicate him/herself if authorized by a physician and parent.

Sincerely,

_____	_____
(Physician's signature)	(Parent's signature)
_____	_____
Address	Address
_____	_____
City, State, Zip	City, State, Zip
_____	_____
Telephone	Telephone

YOUR SCHOOL'S RESPONSIBILITY

When it comes to dealing with allergies at school, it can help you to know what your school's responsibilities are with regard to your care. That way, you can know what to expect and what to ask for if you aren't getting it. If you have a severe, life-threatening allergy (such as to food or medications), your school is responsible for the following: First, your school is responsible for including you in all school activities. As a student with allergies, you should not be excluded from any activity based solely on your allergy. They are also responsible for reviewing the health records submitted by your parents and your physician; following all federal, state, and district laws and regulations that govern sharing your medication information; and prohibiting the allergen from entering any classroom where you are sitting. Tables should be washed with soap and water in the morning if an event has taken place in the classroom the night before. Your school should also ensure that all staff members who work with you on a regular basis understand your allergy, can recognize the symptoms of your allergy, and know what to do in the event of an attack.

In addition, your school should coordinate with the school nurse to make sure all medications are appropriately stored, and they should keep an emergency medication kit (Epipen or Twinject) that contains your physician's prescribed dose on hand. Beyond that, your school is responsible for making sure that students who come in contact with you practice proper hand washing techniques before and after handling or consuming food; designating school personnel who are properly trained to give medication; and identifying a core team of people to work with you and your parents to develop a prevention plan. This team can include (but is not limited to) your school nurse, principal, school food service and nutrition manager/director, and counselor (if available). The school should also work with staff to eliminate the use of allergens in your meals, educational tools, or arts and crafts projects, and administrators and teachers should practice food allergy action plans before an allergic reaction occurs to ensure the effectiveness of the plans.

With respect to transportation, your school should make sure that the school bus driver training program includes what to do if an allergic reaction occurs (if you ride the bus); they should recommend that all school bus drivers have a communication device (such as a cell phone or walkie-talkie) in the event of an emergency; and a no-eating policy should be enforced on all school buses. Your school should also discuss field trips with you and your parents beforehand to decide appropriate strategies for managing your allergies on the trip.

Overall, your school should be prepared to handle a reaction and to make sure there is a staff member who is properly trained to administer medications available to you at all times. They should take any threats or harassment against you seriously, and they should review your action plan with you, your parents, the core team members, and your physician after you have experienced an allergy attack.

WHAT YOU NEED TO KNOW

> Your allergies may flare up at school because classrooms can be a breeding ground for allergens. If a school is poorly ventilated and damp (which many are), allergy-causing mold will grow there. Guinea pigs and white mice add a nice educational component to science classes, but they are also full of allergens.

> No matter what your allergy, to avoid it at school, the best thing you can do as you start a new school year is have an allergy treatment plan in place *before* the first day.

> Before your first day, set up a meeting between you, a parent, your homeroom teacher, school nurse, cafeteria staff, and school principal. At the meeting, discuss your allergies or asthma, which medications you need and when, and any special instructions, such as dietary limitations or avoiding certain substances.

> Remember that *you* are your best first line of defense. You have the power to protect yourself at school by carrying your medications at all times and by doing what you can to make sure your environment is as allergen-free as possible.

- If you need to carry epinephrine (EpiPen or Twinject) because you have a life-threatening allergy to food or insect stings, recognize that you are legally permitted to carry the medication in your purse, pocket, or backpack.
- In addition to your teachers and bus driver, if it is severe, make sure all your friends and classmates are aware of your allergy.
- During an allergy attack at school, always err on the side of caution. If you are able, give yourself an epinephrine (EpiPen or Twinject) shot the moment you start to experience symptoms.
- If you have a severe food allergy, do not trade food with classmates; do not eat anything that is known to contain your allergen or that contains unknown ingredients; notify an adult immediately if you think you ate something that contains the food to which you are allergic; and consider sitting at a "peanut-free" or "shellfish-free" table to minimize your chances of exposure.
- If you suspect you are allergic to something in your environment at school, first, if you haven't already, visit an allergist, immunologist, or your family doctor and explain your symptoms.
- Whenever you travel on field trips, do some preparation. You and the chaperone should carry a copy of your allergy action plan and/or emergency plan, which should include the name and phone number of the nearest hospital. If your allergy is life-threatening, the school nurse may accompany you on the trip.

7

Allergies and Your Social Life

Whether it is with your clothes, your hair, or your attitude, as a teen, you probably go to great lengths to fit in with your friends and peers. Regretfully, many teenagers' desire to fit in puts them at risk. A study published in the *Journal of Allergy and Clinical Immunology* showed that many teenagers with food allergies are being careless. Conducted by Dr. Scott Sicherer and Hugh Sampson of the Mt. Sinai School of Medicine, and Food Allergy and Anaphylaxis Network (FAAN) founder and CEO, Anne Muñoz-Furlong, the study surveyed 174 teens between the ages of 13 and 21 and found that a significant number of those questioned admitted to potentially life-threatening activities with regard to their food allergies, particularly when they were out with friends. According to the study, only 61 percent of teens said they carried their epinephrine all the time, 94 percent reported carrying it when they were traveling, 43 percent said they carried it when they were participating in sports or other activities, 53 percent reported carrying it when they were wearing tight clothing, and 61 percent said they brought it with them to school dances. Perhaps the most alarming finding from the study was that 54 percent (more than half!) of teens with serious food allergies admitted to eating potentially unsafe foods from time to time.

Why are so many of these teens taking these potentially life-threatening risks? Because it is so important for teenagers to fit in with friends, they don't have direct parental supervision from their parents for the first time in their lives, and they have the false notion that

90

they are invincible. These reasons definitely do not make this kind of risk-taking behavior okay. For teens with food allergies, taking even a bite of a food to which they are allergic can be deadly. Because a separate study found that 69 percent of people who died from food allergy reactions were between the ages of 12 and 21, the bulk of the risk-takers when it comes to food allergies are in their teenage years. This does not have to mean you, however. As a mature and responsible teen, you can—and should—take control of food allergies or other allergies you may suffer from to keep yourself as safe and healthy as possible.

The good news is that you can take control of your allergy and/or asthma and have a relatively normal social life at the same time. With the correct information and planning tools from your allergist and the right attitude and imagination, you can stay overnight at friends' houses, eat out at restaurants, go away to college, and do many other things that nonallergic teens do.

THE EMOTIONAL TOLL OF ALLERGIES

It is no secret that teenagers with allergies have it tougher than teenagers without allergies. On top of the other pressures that all teens deal with, such as the physical changes of puberty, making new friends in middle and high school, and striving to wear the right clothes, you have to manage your allergy. During these pivotal years in your life when you are becoming an adult and spending more time in coffee shops, malls, and diners with friends, the last thing you want is to stick out or be stifled because you have allergies or asthma. You don't want to be marooned at a designated table at lunch with "safe" foods while your friends munch on ice cream cones covered in peanuts. You don't want to sit out during gym class while your classmates play basketball, and you don't want to carry cumbersome medications in your purse or backpack. However, to keep yourself safe, as a teen with allergies, there are some precautions you simply have to take despite some slight social sacrifices.

Because you have to take some extra measures, you may feel stressed out and depressed from time to time, and that is normal and expected. Allergists frequently deal with teenagers who come to them complaining of anxiety, sadness, and depression. These feelings are the result not only of the physical discomfort but also of the stress their allergy or asthma has put upon their friends and family. A teenager with eczema will experience embarrassment because of his rash, discomfort because of the itching, and emotional upheaval after watching his mother and father obsess about his condition. At the same time, this boy may struggle with socializing and dating at school, stress over having to carry his daily medication, and worry over being exposed to something that will aggravate his itchy rash. It is a tough situation for him and for every teenager with allergies or asthma, and it can take a toll on self-esteem and well-being. Again, this is not to make you feel as though you are socially doomed as a teen with allergies—you most certainly are not. It is simply to let you

Eczema and Your Social Life

When it flares up at its worst, eczema can be detrimental to your social life. The good news about eczema is that it usually clears up by the time you reach 25; so if you are in your late teens, you are in the home stretch. The bad news is that your late teens and early 20s can be some of the prime socializing years of your life, so to ease the physical and social stress of eczema, here are some actions you can take:

➤ If you wear makeup, be choosy about your brands. Look for makeup that is free of fragrances and dyes—it will make flare-ups less likely. Your dermatologist will be able to suggest brands that are less likely to aggravate the condition.

➤ Get moving. Because sweat can irritate your skin, you may be tempted to skip working out, but exercise is a great way to reduce the stress that can come along with eczema. To lessen the burning and irritation, choose activities that keep your skin cool and dry while you are working out, such as walking and bike riding.

➤ Get involved. Although you may feel like hiding away, socializing is one of the best things you can do for your skin because it will get your mind off the itching. There may be certain activities that cause your eczema to flare up, such as swimming in a heavily chlorinated pool. If that's the case, simply avoid doing those after-school activities and ask your friends if you can do something else; if they are true friends, they will be happy to oblige.

know that you are not alone in your feelings and to urge you to share them with your parents, friends, and/or allergist.

FOOD ALLERGIES AND YOUR SOCIAL LIFE

Perhaps the most alarming allergy when it comes to socializing with friends is a food allergy. While nasal and skin allergies can dampen your social life, they are not dangerous. If you make the wrong decision with a serious food allergy, however, it could be fatal.

One of the most threatening places for you if you have a severe food allergy is unfortunately one of the most popular hangouts for teens—the ice cream shop. With all the nut-containing toppings, such as M&Ms, peanuts, and toffee, combined with the high possibility of cross-contamination, ice cream shops are a real danger zone. The ice cream shop may be one place you simply have to avoid if you have a serious food allergy. If your friends insist on getting ice cream, to avoid feeling deprived, swing by a convenience store for a fudge pop or another "safe" ice cream food and wait outside while your friends order. Ask them to avoid anything with nuts and be careful about getting too close to or kissing any of them in the event that one of their ice cream treats accidentally got hit with some nuts or another allergen.

Beyond the ice cream shop, if you have a food allergy, you also know it can be tough to eat in other types of restaurants. What is supposed to be a pleasurable experience causes stress and anxiety, and with good reason. A survey conducted by the Food Allergy and Anaphylaxis Network revealed that almost all people with food allergies report having had an allergic reaction to a food served in a restaurant. The most frequently expressed concerns of people surveyed are that there will be cross-contamination in the kitchen, that the staff won't take their food allergies seriously, or that there will be a lack of awareness or concern by the restaurant with regard to their allergies. These fears are not unjustified, but if you take some stringent precautions, you can enjoy eating out as much as your nonallergic friends and family members.

First, when you plan to eat out, choose a restaurant with simple menu items. Hibachi restaurants that cook multiple meals on the same grill at the same time are definitely out for you, as are Thai restaurants, bakeries, Chinese restaurants, and other restaurants that stir-fry and cook with a lot of nuts. Thai restaurants especially cook with peanuts a great deal. Food cooked in woks may open the risk of cross-contamination. Once you have chosen a suitable restaurant, ask to see a menu a few days ahead of time, so you can think about your options. That way, if the menu doesn't contain any safe choices, you can call and ask if they will make you a special meal that is void of all of your allergens. This preplanning will prevent the embarrassment of having to ask numerous questions in front of your friends, and it will save you the discomfort of having to go hungry.

When you eat at friends' houses, the situation can be a little stickier. You don't want to seem like a high-maintenance guest or appear ungrateful if you cannot eat a meal you are served, but you shouldn't be shy. True friends and their parents will be sympathetic to your allergy and happy to make you something you can safely eat. Or, if you aren't comfortable getting a special meal, simply eat the meat and plain vegetables (provided you are not allergic to these things) and skip the sauces and side dishes that may contain hidden allergens. If you are unsure of whether a vegetable or meat has been marinated in a sauce that could potentially contain an allergen, don't be afraid to ask the host or hostess. The same rules apply to beverages—if you aren't sure of the contents of a beverage, ask or skip it and stick with water.

Prepacked or picnic lunches on field trips or day outings provide challenges as well. Depending on what you are allergic to, stick with plain, safe foods, such as fresh rolls, chicken, roast beef, lettuce, tomatoes, and carrots. No matter where you plan to eat, if it is away from home, it is a good rule of thumb to have a snack before you go in case any of the menu items are off limits for you.

On the occasions when you travel with family and friends, you may not be able to be as controlled with your eating. The secret is to plan your trip carefully. For a road trip, pack plenty of safe foods in a cooler. If you will be staying in a hotel, book your overnight accommodation in a room that has facilities for cooking your own food, and order meals ahead of time. When you fly, pack enough food for the flight *and* for your first day at your destination in your carry-on bag, and avoid airline meals unless the airline staff knows of your allergy and assures you that the meal contains none of the foods to which you are allergic. If you have a severe peanut allergy, tell the staff when you book your flight—they will make sure no peanuts are served or eaten on the plane. Some airlines at the time of this publication are resistant to changes. For additional advice on how to handle food allergies, see Chapter 8.

CARRYING MEDICATIONS IN SOCIAL SITUATIONS

Depending on your personality, you may despise having to carry allergy medication, an EpiPen or Twinject, or an inhaler wherever

Real-Life Scenario

One important topic to keep in mind if you are an older teen with aller-gies is dating. As the following real-life scenario shows, if you have a severe food allergy and are not especially careful when you are dating, it can have dire consequences.

Jaime, a 19-year-old patient with a peanut allergy, went on a date with Kyle, her boyfriend of a few months. Before their date, Kyle remembered that he had eaten a peanut butter sandwich for lunch, so being aware of Jaime's allergy, he brushed his teeth and rinsed out his mouth with mouthwash before heading over to her apartment.

Jaime made dinner for Kyle—peanut free, of course—and then they set-tled down to watch a movie on the couch. They started kissing and Jaime asked, "you didn't have any peanuts today, did you?" Kyle replied that he had had some for lunch, but that he had thoroughly brushed, flossed, and mouthwashed before he came over. Knowing that the anaphylactic reaction would kick in quickly if there were indeed still peanuts in Kyle's mouth, and also realizing that her EpiPen was just a few feet away, Jaime decided to take her chances and continue with the kissing.

After a few minutes, Jaime was fine, so she knew Kyle's mouth was peanut-free. One thing led to another and they ended up becoming inti-mate. Right afterward, Jaime's throat started closing—she was having a reaction! She reached for the EpiPen beside her bed, injected herself, and after a few minutes, she was fine; but she was confused—why had she had an anaphylactic attack?! It turns out that although there were no peanuts left in Kyle's mouth or saliva, there were some remaining in his body, enough to come out in his semen and cause a reaction in Jaime.

The lesson here is that you can never be too careful as a teenager with a severe food allergy. Even if you take extra precautions to avoid the foods to which you are allergic—and as this story illustrates, even if your date does—you can still have a reaction. Talk to your date openly and honestly about your allergy, and make sure he or she washes his or her hands, brushes his or her teeth, flosses, and uses mouthwash before kissing you, and also be sure to avoid intercourse or use con-doms if there is even the slightest chance that your date was exposed to your allergen in the last 24 hours, and always carry your EpiPen or Twinject with you wherever you go.

you go; you might feel indifferent about the situation; or you may actually enjoy it because it makes you feel in control, but personality aside, if you have an allergy or asthma that requires medication, particularly if it is emergency medication, you *must* carry it, no matter how socially awkward it may make you feel. Here are some things you can do to make carrying allergy medication a little less of a social burden.

First, realize the importance of your medication. Depending on the severity of your allergy or asthma, carrying the proper medication with you literally can mean the difference between life and death. At the time, it may seem more important to wear the tight-fitting jeans without worrying about the bulge of an EpiPen, but if you suffer an attack, that fashion statement could be deadly. At this point in your life, you may feel invincible, but you are not, and you are much more vulnerable than your nonallergic friends.

Consider cargo pants. Luckily, these days both tight-fitting and baggy pants with pockets are in style for guys and girls. If you must carry medication and you do not (or would rather not) carry a purse or backpack, cargo pants, cargo shorts, or even cargo skirts can be the perfect solution. Not only will they provide plenty of room for an EpiPen or Twinject, cargo pants, shorts, and skirts usually have Velcro or snaps on the pockets to help ensure that your medication won't fall out.

Carry your allergy or asthma emergency plan too. Since cargo pants, shorts, and skirts have multiple pockets, you will have a place for your allergy action or emergency plan as well. With this, you will have the tools necessary to instruct others on how to help you in the event that you can't give medication to yourself. If you are carrying an EpiPen or Twinject, it is a good idea to include the directions for administering these medications on your emergency plan.

If your allergy or asthma requires that you take medication regularly, do not miss a dose. When you're caught up in the moment socializing with friends, it can be easy to forget to take your medication, but it is no less important. So do something to remind yourself. Set the alarm on your cell phone to go off at the time you need your meds, or ask a friend or family member to call you as a reminder. Remembering to take your medications will allow you to enjoy social outings without symptoms, ensuring that you have the most fun possible.

DEALING WITH ALLERGIES IN COLLEGE

At the end of your teenage years, going away to college is likely to be at the forefront in your mind. College is a time of great educational and social transition, and if you have allergies or asthma, it is also a time when you will have to be particularly careful. Studies have shown that students in their early 20s are at the height of impulsive decision making—a practice that will not mesh well with a severe allergy. In college, you will be exposed to new plants, pollens, insects, and molds; you will have to share kitchens and pitchers; and you will have to navigate meal plans and dining halls—all without the constant support of your parents. At the same time, college will be one of the most exciting times of your life, and you have just as much of a right to enjoy it as your nonallergic classmates.

As a teenager with allergies, college will be a crossroads of sorts. If you are moving away from your allergist and you take allergy shots,

The Kissing Study

In 2006, a study conducted at the Elliot and Roslyn Jaffe Food Allergy Institute, Division of Allergy and Immunology, Department of Pediatrics, Mount Sinai School of Medicine and published in the *Journal of Allergy and Clinical Immunology*, investigated how long peanut allergen stays in a person's saliva after they have eaten it. Researchers asked 10 people to eat a peanut butter sandwich and then collected saliva samples from their mouths at different times, including after they had brushed their teeth and used mouthwash. The results were surprising: Immediately after eating the sandwich, all of the participants (those who had rinsed, brushed, and done neither) had measurable levels of peanut allergen in their mouths. One hour after eating the sandwich, four people had detectable levels of the allergen in their mouths, and four and a half hours after the sandwiches were eaten, none of the participants had detectable levels in their saliva. The study shows that people who eat any form of peanuts must wait several hours and brush their teeth before kissing someone with a peanut allergy. And as Jaime's story above illustrates, even when the mouth is clean, other precautions must be taken.

you will have to decide whether or not to continue them. You will have to make the decision of whether to live on campus in a dorm, in which case you will eat in the dining hall, or off campus in an apartment, where you will have to share a kitchen with roommates—a tough choice if you have a severe food allergy. Or, if you are nervous about being exposed to your allergen(s), you may decide to request a single room, an option most colleges and universities offer to students with serious allergies. When you enter the big, new, autonomous world of college, you will need to develop your own safety and decision making strategies.

A bit of good news is that because there are so many teenagers with allergies entering colleges and universities these days, some schools are starting to make some encouraging advancements. For example, a few schools have eliminated nuts from dining hall menus and are offering allergy-friendly foods, and others are hiring emergency response teams to carry an EpiPen or Twinject and administer medications in the event a student has an allergy attack.

Since most colleges and universities have been relatively slow to adapt to students with allergies, the bulk of the responsibility lies in your hands. Given all the other new responsibilities on your shoulders as a college student, taking steps to avoid an allergy attack can be overwhelming, but it is vital. Here are some specific actions you can take to better protect yourself.

A month or two before classes start:

> Inform the college or university you will be attending about your allergies and get as much information as possible.
> Contact residence life or student life and inform them of your allergy and the medications you require, both on a daily basis and in the event of an emergency.
> Talk to campus security and discuss the protocol in the event that you suffer a reaction. On some campuses, students are requested to call campus security during an emergency; on others, students are asked to dial 911. Knowing what you should do ahead of time will help you eliminate confusion in the face of a sudden attack.
> Meet with your college or university's health center to inquire about the nearest hospital, discuss emergency procedures, and find out which medications they carry.
> Ask your doctor to provide a letter documenting your allergy restrictions, symptoms, instructions for medications, and procedures to follow to treat a reaction. The Food Allergy & Anaphylaxis Network's College Food Allergy Action Plan is a great tool for recording this information (see Chapter 6).

➤ Find an allergist near your school. If you are going to a college or university that is more than an hour away from your home, you will have to switch allergists. Ask your present physician to recommend an allergist in the area where your school is located.

➤ Schedule a meeting or phone conversation with the director of food service and inquire about meal plans, ask if the staff is trained to deal with severe allergic reactions and, if necessary, request that they prepare your meals in advance.

➤ Beyond dining halls, ask about food served in other locations. Many universities have fast food and other restaurants and snack stands on campus, and food is often served at sporting events. If you plan on eating at these places, visit them before classes start and ask for ingredients lists.

➤ Consider a single room in a newer residence. Newer dorm rooms are more likely to have tile or hardwood flooring than dust-mite filled carpeting, and a single room will prevent exposure to allergens brought in by a roommate.

Once school starts:

➤ In the dining hall, avoid foods that are at a high risk for cross-contamination, such as baked goods, ice cream toppings, and cereals.

➤ Be sure to carry your medical insurance card with you at all times.

➤ If one is not provided, think about buying a combination microwave/refrigerator for your dorm room so you can prepare your own meals.

➤ If you have a roommate, talk to him or her about your allergy. Teach your roommate to recognize the signs of an allergy attack, and if you carry an EpiPen or Twinject, show him or her how to administer the medication in the event of an emergency.

➤ Request that your roommate avoid eating the food(s) to which you are allergic in your dorm room. If he or she resists, be extra careful to avoid cross-contamination and wash counters and utensils thoroughly.

➤ If you have a food allergy, make several copies of your Food Allergy Action Plan and post it in your dining hall, next to the phone in your dorm room, and in your Resident Adviser (RA)'s room.

➤ If you live near your college or university, consider commuting rather than living on campus. You may feel slightly restricted socially, but if you have a life-threatening allergy, it's better to be safe than sorry.

▸ Know which situations you must avoid. If your friends are going to hang out at a bar that serves peanuts and you have a peanut allergy, for example, you will probably have to skip it. Part of being a responsible young adult with allergies is realizing whether a social situation is worth the risk.

▸ If you have a severe food allergy, tell your professors, and ask them to request that students refrain from eating that food in class.

▸ If you need emergency medication or an inhaler, carry it with you at *all* times, and be sure to wear your Medic Alert ID bracelet if you require one. It may seem like a pain to lug an EpiPen or Twinject to a fraternity party, but luck may have it that the time you are without your medication, you suffer an attack. So never leave it at home.

▸ Keep your wits about you. If you drink too much or take recreational drugs, you will be more likely to practice poor judgment and accidentally expose yourself to your allergen(s).

WHAT YOU NEED TO KNOW

▸ If you have a severe food allergy, you must be extremely careful in social situations. For teens with food allergies, taking even a bite of a food to which they are allergic can be deadly.

▸ Having allergies doesn't have to spoil your social life. With the correct information and planning tools from your allergist and the right attitude and imagination, you can stay overnight at friends' houses, eat out at restaurants, go away to college, and do many other things that nonallergic teens do.

▸ However, to keep yourself safe, as a teen with allergies, there are some precautions you simply have to take despite some slight social sacrifices.

▸ Because you have to take some extra measures, you may feel stressed out and depressed from time to time, and that is normal and expected.

▸ Be extra careful in restaurants. A survey conducted by the Food Allergy & Anaphylaxis Network revealed that almost all people with food allergies report having had an allergic reaction to a food served in a restaurant.

▸ Taking care of your allergies is important when you travel. For example, for a road trip, pack plenty of safe foods in a cooler. If you will be staying in a hotel, book your overnight accommodation in a room that has facilities for cooking your own food, and order meals ahead of time.

Surprising Facts about Allergies

- ▶ Cat allergies are one of the most common allergies. Almost 10 million people are allergic to cats.

- ▶ As gross as it sounds, dust mites are attracted to and feed on flakes of your skin.

- ▶ Ninety percent of all food allergies are caused by eight main foods: milk, soy, eggs, wheat, peanuts, tree nuts, fish, and shellfish.

- ▶ 150 to 200 people die of food anaphylaxis each year, and children age 10 to 19 are at the greatest risk.

- ▶ Latex allergy is responsible for more than 200 cases of anaphylaxis each year, and 10 percent of health-care workers have latex allergies.

- ▶ Each year, nearly 100 Americans die from insect stings.

- ▶ Allergies cost the country nearly $7 billion per year.

▶ Realize the importance of your medication. Depending on the severity of your allergy or asthma, carrying the proper medication with you, such as an EpiPen or Twinject, literally can mean the difference between life and death. If your allergy or asthma requires that you take medication regularly, do not miss a dose.

▶ If you plan to go away to college, take some precautionary steps with respect to your allergies. For example, inform the college or university you will be attending about your allergies and get as much information as possible; contact residence life or student life administrators and inform them of your allergy and the medications you require, both on a daily basis and in the event of an emergency; find an allergist near your school; in the dining hall, avoid foods that are at a high risk for cross-contamination, such as baked goods, ice cream toppings, and cereals; and keep your wits about you. If you drink too much or take recreational drugs, you will be more likely to practice poor judgment and accidentally expose yourself to your allergen(s).

8

It's in What You Eat: Food Allergies

For Brenton Schively, age 16, neglecting to ask about the ingredients in a cookie cost him his life. Brenton was at a friend's house and innocently took a cookie from a bowl on the kitchen table. He immediately felt a tingling in his mouth, called his mom, and took an antihistamine. An hour later, he was dead.

Brenton's story is not meant to scare teens with food allergies; rather, it is intended to alert them to the dangers of neglecting to be vigilant. Most of the deaths from food allergies occur in teenagers, an indication that teens with food allergies are not being as careful as they should be. In a Web survey answered by 174 teenagers with food allergies, 44 percent admitted to occasionally eating a small amount of a food known to contain their allergens, and 42 percent said they ate a food in a label that said it "may contain" the food to which they were allergic. Another study conducted at the National Jewish Medical and Research Center in Denver, Colorado, and Mount Sinai School of Medicine in New York showed that few teens ask about ingredients in foods they order in restaurants and that of those who had accidentally died from a food allergy, 58 percent were between the age of 13 and 30.

A food allergy may be particularly frustrating in your teenage years, when thoughts of dating and college overshadow the importance of remembering to read food labels. Becoming a teenager no doubt comes with increasing independence, but it is important to remember that with independence comes great responsibility, especially if you are a teen with a food allergy. In addition to playing sports, attending school dances, and studying for tests, one of your jobs is to closely watch out for yourself. You must be careful about every food that goes in your mouth or into the mouth of someone you are going to kiss or be close to. If your allergy is particularly severe, you will have to be mindful of foods you touch or breathe in, too. Food allergies differ from other types of allergies in that even a tiny amount of the food—small enough to float through the air—can be fatal; with other allergies, such as those to dust or mold, the severity of the attack is usually proportionate to the amount of the allergen a person has encountered.

Overall, having a food allergy does not mean you can't do all the things you love; you just need to take the right precautions. This chapter will give you information to help you better understand and manage your food allergy, including what causes it, the symptoms, the dangers, and what you can do to keep yourself healthy and alive.

THE CAUSE OF FOOD ALLERGIES

Although 13 to 18 percent of people in the United States claim to have a food allergy, only 2 percent actually do. Why the discrepancy? People often confuse food allergies with food intolerances, such as those to *lactose* or wheat, because allergies and intolerances sometimes cause similar symptoms, like stomach upset. Unlike food allergies, however, intolerances are rarely dangerous. In addition, people may mistake any adverse reaction to a food as being allergic in nature. For example, spoiled fish can cause a rash that is neither an allergy nor an intolerance. All symptoms should be reviewed with one's physician or health-care professional.

True food allergies result when your immune system mistakenly believes something you have eaten is harmful to your body. In attempt to protect itself from the food, your immune system produces IgE antibodies—special proteins the body makes in response to substances it thinks are harmful. These IgE antibodies then cause allergy cells in your body called mast cells to release symptom-causing chemicals into your bloodstream, including histamine, leukotrienes, and prostaglandins. These chemicals, particularly histamine, cause a reaction in your eyes, nose, throat, gastrointestinal tract, or skin. Then, the next time you eat that particular food, those antibodies will instantly recognize it and launch another attack—probably a worse one.

When you develop an allergy to dust, pollen, or a certain food, you are actually reacting to the proteins in these substances. Allergic reactions are actually left over from the days when our bodies fought parasites, and they are rich in protein. So when your body encounters an egg white omelet or a piece of cheese, it may confuse these benign proteins with those in threatening bugs.

It is also thought that allergies, including food allergies, are partially the result of modernization. There are more food-allergic children, teens, and adults than ever before, suggesting that something in the environment may be triggering the problem. Some modern inventions that may be contributing include the shoe, energy-efficient housing, and antibiotics that fight germs. All three advancements have kept people protected from invaders that they previously encountered on a regular basis. As a result, our immune systems are revved up with nothing to fight, forcing them to react to foods and other allergens as they used to react to parasites.

In addition to environmental changes, food allergies are influenced by your genes. If one of your parents has a food allergy, your chances of having one yourself are one in three. If both of your parents have food allergies, your odds rise to seven in 10. And some studies have shown that when mothers breast-feed their babies, the breast milk helps protect them against major food allergens; so if you were not breast-fed, you may have inadvertently been put at a higher risk.

Unfortunately, just because you are food allergy-free today doesn't mean that will always be the case. While people are indeed born with a genetic predisposition to allergies, some don't develop symptoms until adulthood. Researchers think that the more frequently you are exposed to an allergen, the more antibodies build up until one day they are released in the form of an attack. Once that first reaction occurs, you will have one each time you are exposed to the allergen.

SYMPTOMS OF FOOD ALLERGIES

With some food allergies, such as peanut and shellfish allergies, the reaction can be life-threatening. As experienced by Brenton Schively, a food allergy can cause a severe reaction called anaphylaxis, which sets in in as little as five to 15 minutes and leads to itchiness, hives, breathing problems, a sense of impending doom, a drop in blood pressure, a decreased blood flow, especially to the brain, heart, and lungs, and in some cases, death. The reaction has been likened to a snowball rolling down a mountain—it gets worse as it progresses. When someone experiences a severe food allergy that results in anaphylaxis, immediate emergency treatment is necessary. This treatment includes the medication epinephrine, a drug that increases blood pressure. (Epinephrine is available in portable injection kits under the brand names EpiPen and Twinject.) If you or someone you know has a severe allergic reaction to a food, you should call 911 immediately and administer a dose of epinephrine in the meantime.

There is strong scientific evidence to back up the need for epinephrine in the treatment of food allergies: Hugh A. Sampson, M.D., a leading expert in food allergies, did a study on anaphylactic reactions together with his colleagues at Johns Hopkins University School of Medicine in Baltimore in the early 1990s on 13 children who had severe food allergies. He found that children who suffer

How to Tell the Difference between a Food Intolerance and a Food Allergy

Although between 13 and 18 percent of the population claim to have a food allergy, only about 2 percent actually do. This doesn't mean the remaining 11 to 16 percent are imagining their symptoms, however; they are just misdiagnosing them. This group of people actually has what's called a food intolerance, which differs from a food allergy in a few different ways.

With food allergy, the reaction begins in a person's immune system. The immune system falsely identifies the food as an invader and releases antibodies to fight it off. The most common allergic reactions occur in the mouth, digestive tract, skin, and airways. With a food intolerance, on the other hand, the problem lies within a person's metabolism. When someone has an intolerance to the lactose in milk, for example, he experiences diarrhea and vomiting after eating a dairy product because he is deficient in the intestinal enzyme lactase, which is necessary to digest milk sugar. Other food intolerances that are on the rise include those to aspartame, an artificial sweetener; monosodium glutamate (MSG), a flavor-enhancer; and tartrazine, also called FD&C yellow number 5, a food coloring.

Both food allergies and food intolerances will probably require that you stay away from the offending food, but it is important that you get a proper diagnosis. If you suspect you have a food allergy, the only way to find out if it is an allergy in the true sense of the word is to visit your family physician or an allergist.

from anaphylaxis should be observed in a hospital or medical center for at least three to four hours after the reaction, and that epinephrine should definitely be prescribed and kept available to all people with severe food allergies.

Other symptoms of food allergies may vary based on the food eaten, but in general, some of the first signs can include a runny nose, an itchy skin rash, or tingling in the tongue, lips, or throat. Additional reactions may include swelling in the throat or other parts of the body, eczema, abdominal pain, diarrhea or vomiting, dizziness, and wheezing. Some people start to experience symptoms within seconds of eating a trigger food; others don't notice them for several hours.

DEALING WITH FOOD ALLERGIES

If you have a food allergy, whether it is mild, moderate, or severe, the only way to deal with it is to avoid the trigger food(s) and to be on the lookout for symptoms. If your allergy is severe, as little as one fifth to one five-thousandth of a teaspoon of the offender may cause death; therefore, you may not only have to avoid eating the food, you may have to steer clear of touching the food, refrain from entering a room or area where the food has been, or stay away from people who have eaten the food. Make sure that your family, friends, and acquaintances all know about your allergy, so they can alert you to danger foods and help get you medical attention in the event of an emergency. Also be careful of cross-contamination in your home, which can happen on knives or in the toaster.

One way to avoid your trigger food is to carefully read labels. As of January 2006, food manufacturers must state on labels if a food contains one of the eight most common food allergens—milk, eggs, fish, shellfish, peanuts and tree nuts, wheat, and soy. For example, if the hydrogenated vegetable protein in a food comes from peanuts, the label should say so. Despite the recent improvements in labeling, you should still be educated on hidden allergens in foods. Dr. Sampson's study revealed that six deaths occurred because either the child or his or her parent was unaware that a certain food contained an allergen because it was listed under a different name.

In addition, you should take the following precautions, no matter what your specific trigger food:

▸ Always be careful about eating food in the school cafeteria.
▸ Eat off of a napkin to avoid potentially contaminated surfaces.

> Ask about ingredients *every time* you purchase a food or eat a food in a restaurant or at a friend's house.
> Eat lunch with friends who know about your food allergy and are prepared to help and/or treat you in the event of an attack.
> If you feel like you might be suffering a reaction, tell those around you immediately.
> Identify the source of the food by speaking to the cook or chef and asking her or him what is in it.

An estimated 12 million people in the United States have food allergies, but those allergies are only due to eight different foods. The most common food allergens, which cause 90 percent of food allergies, are milk, eggs, wheat, soy, peanuts and tree nuts, fish, and shellfish. Although it is thought that people with food allergies are allergic to many foods, most react to fewer than four food allergens. To give you a better understanding of your specific food allergy(s) and their symptoms, here is an overview.

MILK ALLERGY

Milk allergy is a tough one. From ice cream to pizza to cheeseburgers, it is in almost all foods that teenagers love. Luckily, milk allergy is more common in children because it is often the result of an immature digestive system that can't handle the milk proteins—80 percent of kids outgrow milk allergy by the time they reach age six. Therefore, if you were allergic to milk when you were a child, chances are, you're over it. If your milk allergy has persisted, however, it is probably fairly severe.

Milk allergy should not be confused with lactose intolerance, a condition that involves difficulty digesting the sugars in milk. Lactose intolerance falls into the category of a food sensitivity and produces bloating, cramping, gas, diarrhea, and nausea. A true milk allergy, on the other hand, is an allergic reaction to one or more of the proteins in milk, and it will cause hives, headaches, vomiting, and/or trouble breathing within minutes to hours of drinking milk or eating a dairy product. Rarely, people with milk allergy will have an anaphylactic reaction after ingesting it. Most reactions last less than a day.

Because milk and dairy products are found in so many foods, you may want to work with a registered dietitian to develop an eating plan that offers nutritious and tasty alternatives to dairy. Luckily, many nondairy foods, such as orange juice and cereals, are now fortified with calcium, so it is easy for you to get enough of this important mineral. Vegan foods, which you can find at health food stores, are made without dairy. For a direct cow's milk substitute, you can drink rice milk or soy milk (but not goat's milk, which contains a similar protein to the cow form). In place of ice cream, you can eat sorbet, dairy-free pudding, ice pops, or soy or rice-based frozen desserts. For baking, milk substitutes work just as well as the real thing, and dairy-free margarine makes a fine alternative to butter on toast or a bagel. Also watch out for fried foods; the batter could contain milk, or the food may have been fried in oil used to fry something containing dairy.

As with other allergies, you should check the labels of all foods you eat to make sure they don't contain milk. Since labels often use a different name for milk or milk products, you should be educated on the different milk terms. Here are some of the most common names for milk or milk protein on labels. For maximum safety, carry this list with you at all times:

Artificial butter flavor
Butter
Butter fat
Buttermilk
Caseinates (ammonium, calcium, magnesium, potassium, sodium)
Cheese
Cottage cheese
Curds
Cream
Custard or pudding
Ghee (clarified butter used in Indian cooking)
Half and half
Hydrolysates (casein, milk protein, protein, whey, whey protein)
Lactalbumin
Lactalbumin phosphate
Lactoglobulin
Milk (derivative, protein, solids, malted, condensed, evaporated, dry, whole, low-fat, nonfat, skim)
Sour cream
Sour cream solids
Whey (delactosed, demineralized, protein, concentrate)
Yogurt

Dining Out with Food Allergies

For people with severe food allergies, eating out at restaurants can be more stressful than fun. To make it more tolerable, do the following:

▶ Let the waitstaff know about your allergy and don't be afraid to ask detailed questions about menu items.

▶ Before you order a food, ask if it contains your trigger food(s).

▶ Order the simplest foods on the menu.

▶ Ask the waitstaff if the food you plan to order has been prepared with or near the trigger food; if they do not know, ask the kitchen staff. If you aren't sure, choose another "safe" menu item.

▶ If you have an allergy that may lead to anaphylaxis, avoid Thai, Chinese, Mexican, Indonesian, African, and Vietnamese restaurants and dishes—they may be prepared in a kitchen (or in a way) where foods may come in contact with peanuts, nuts, eggs, seafood, or another allergen.

PEANUT AND NUT ALLERGY

Peanut and nut allergies are among the most common food allergies. There are two main problems with peanut and nut allergies: 1) They are one of the most serious food allergies, causing life-threatening anaphylaxis in some people, and 2) They make their way into foods and products you would never imagine, such as chili, gravy, ice cream, dog food, bird feed, some cosmetics, and homemade baked goods. While 90 percent of kids with allergies to milk, soy, and other foods will outgrow the allergy by the time they reach their teens, the same is not true for peanut or nut allergies. In fact, only 10 to 20 percent of children with peanut or nut allergies will outgrow the problem, leaving 80 to 90 percent of teenagers with the allergy to continue to deal with it into adulthood.

Peanuts and nuts are distinguished from each other because although peanuts are often thrown into "mixed nut" combinations with tree nuts like almonds, walnuts, pecans and cashews, they are not nuts in the true sense of the word. Peanuts are actually a legume, making them cousins to peas and kidney beans. Both peanuts and nuts cause allergies, however.

People with a nut or peanut allergy may have a mild reaction when they ingest a piece of a nut, and others experience life-threatening anaphylactic reactions. People also differ in how fast their symptoms come on—some folks get a reaction within seconds, and others don't experience symptoms for hours. Most reactions last less than a day, however, and cause the following:

▸ Hives, eczema, and/or redness or swelling around the mouth
▸ Stomach cramps, diarrhea, and/or vomiting
▸ Runny nose, itchy, watery eyes, sneezing, asthma, coughing, and wheezing

As mentioned, in some cases peanuts or nuts lead to a sudden and severe allergic reaction called anaphylaxis. An anaphylactic reaction can involve the respiratory system, gastrointestinal tract, cardiovascular system and skin. Anaphylaxis causes blood pressure to drop, airways to narrow, and the tongue to swell, which leads to serious breathing problems, loss of consciousness, and, in some cases, death. If you have a peanut or nut allergy and experience any of these symptoms, administer your epinephrine injection and get emergency help as soon as possible.

Because a peanut or nut allergy can become so serious so quickly, you must be vigilant about checking the ingredients lists of foods that may contain nuts, asking your friends' parents or restaurant staff members about ingredients in foods you are eating, and avoiding kissing someone who has recently eaten a nut or peanut. Another issue you should keep in mind is cross-contamination, when a food that doesn't include peanuts or nuts gets contaminated because it is processed in a factory that produces nut-containing products. Cross-contamination is a particular risk with chocolate candies, so if your allergy is severe, you should avoid this treat. Or, if you cannot stay away, look for chocolate candies whose manufacturers guarantee that cross-contamination does not take place. To find out which companies promise that their candies are nut- and peanut-free, log on to their Web sites or call the toll-free number on the package.

Some people are so sensitive to nuts and peanuts that they experience a reaction after only breathing in a small particle of a nut. This is why some airlines have stopped serving peanuts, at least when they know someone with a nut allergy is on board. If you fall into this category, you must be *extremely* careful about your surroundings.

In addition to the above tips, if you have a nut or peanut allergy, you should do the following:

- Make sure that you have a Twinject or EpiPen on hand at all times, as well as an over-the-counter antihistamine (antihistamine should be used in addition to an EpiPen or Twinject, not as a replacement).
- Meet with a dietitian to come up with safe meals and snacks.
- Avoid fried foods in restaurants because they may be made with peanut oil or contain hidden nuts or peanuts.
- Always carry a list of the foods you should avoid.
- When you go to other people's houses, parties, and to school, pack your own lunches and snacks so you know they are peanut- and nut-free.
- If your school doesn't already have one, ask to sit at a peanut- and nut-free table at lunch.
- Teach your friends to recognize the symptoms of an anaphylactic reaction as well as how to treat you.
- Be sure that everyone at school—your classmates, coaches, teachers, and principal—knows about your peanut allergy and is ready to act in case you have an anaphylactic reaction.
- Ask your friends, family members, and teachers to wash their hands with soap and water or use hand wipes after meals and snacks.
- Avoid eating at buffets, where people may have put spoons into different bowls.
- Avoid Thai restaurants all together. Many Thai food items have peanuts.

As with other allergies, you should check the labels of all foods you eat to make sure they don't contain peanuts or nuts. Because labels often use a different name for peanuts or nuts, you should be educated on the different terms. Here are some of the most common names for peanuts and nuts on labels. For maximum safety, carry this list with you at all times:

Almonds
Artificial nuts
Beer nuts
Brazil nuts
Cashews

Chestnuts
Cold-pressed, expressed, or expelled peanut oil
Filberts
Gianduja (a creamy mixture of chopped toasted nuts in a high-quality chocolate)
Ground nuts
Hazelnuts
Hickory nuts
Hydrolyzed vegetable protein
Macadamia nuts
Marzipan/almond paste
Mixed nuts
Nougat
Nu-nuts
Nut butters—cashew and almond
Nut oil
Nut paste
Peanut butter
Peanut flour
Pecans
Pine nuts (pignoli, pinion)
Pistachios
Walnuts

Beyond peanut and nut avoidance, which is currently the only way to deal with a peanut allergy, there is some hope on the horizon: the drug *TNX-901,* which may prevent peanut allergies by blocking IgE, the substance that starts the allergic reaction chain, is currently being studied.

WHEAT ALLERGY

Although it is one of the eight most common food allergens, wheat allergy is often confused with wheat intolerance, a condition in which people have trouble digesting a sticky protein called gluten that is found in wheat and other grains. With a true wheat allergy, IgE antibodies are secreted and an allergic reaction occurs within minutes to hours after someone has eaten the food.

Symptoms of wheat allergy range from mild to severe and include congestion, digestion issues (which is why the allergy is so often confused with intolerance), airway inflammation, swelling, itching or irritation in the mouth or throat, and skin reactions. In rare cases, wheat allergy causes life-threatening anaphylaxis. In some people, an allergic reaction to wheat can be brought on by exercising after eating wheat or inhaling flour.

Wheat can be hard to avoid because it is used as an ingredient in numerous foods these days, including some you would never suspect, like ice cream, lunch meats, and sauces. You may want to meet with a registered dietitian to help you develop a safe wheat-free eating plan, and you should check the labels of all foods you eat to make sure they don't contain wheat or wheat products. Because labels often use different names for wheat products, you should educate yourself on the different terms. Here are some of the most common names for wheat on labels. For maximum safety, carry this list with you at all times:

Bread crumbs
Bran
Bulgur
Cereal extract
Cereal
Couscous
Cracker meal
Durum, durum flour
Enriched flour
Farina
Gluten
Graham flour
High-gluten flour
High-protein flour
Kamut
Seitan
Semolina
Spelt (This is often thought to be safe for wheat allergic indi-
    viduals, but it is not true)
Vital gluten
Wheat bran
Wheat germ
Wheat gluten
Wheat malt
Wheat starch
Whole wheat flour
Whole wheat berries

Terms that *may* indicate the presence of wheat:

Soy sauce
Starch (gelatinized, modified, modified food starch, vegetable)
Vegetable gum

FISH AND SHELLFISH ALLERGY

Fish and shellfish allergies are also among the eight most common allergies, and unlike milk and soy allergies, they usually stick with people for life. Like peanut and nut allergies, allergies to fish and shellfish are often severe, bringing on life-threatening anaphylaxis. Just because you are allergic to shellfish doesn't necessarily mean you will definitely also be allergic to fish without shells, but you may be. And some people are allergic to very specific types of shellfish, like shrimp, and not allergic to others, such as clams or scallops. Remember, there are fish with *backbones* like tuna, salmon, etc.; *bivalves* like clams, oysters and mussels; and *arthropods* like lobster, shrimp, and crab. You might be allergic to one class and not to another.

If you have an allergy to fish or shellfish, you will have to make sure you avoid these water dwellers at all costs. One of the most important actions you can take is to stay clear of fried foods (which will benefit your overall health as well); French fries are often cooked in the same oil as fried shrimp and other seafood, and the small amount in the oil is enough to cause a reaction. Obviously, seafood restaurants are not a good choice for you unless they offer numerous other nonseafood menu items and you trust that the kitchen staff won't prepare your meal on a surface that has touched seafood. Another danger zone is a Japanese restaurant, where the chef uses the same grill to prepare shrimp, scallops, chicken, and other dishes. If you or your family chooses to eat at a Japanese restaurant, make sure you clearly explain to the manager and waitstaff that you have a shellfish allergy, and that all grill surfaces will have to be thoroughly cleaned before your meal is prepared.

If you have the potential for anaphylaxis, your doctor will probably want you to carry an EpiPen or Twinject in case of an emergency. If your allergy is less severe, your doctor may instruct you to carry an over-the-counter antihistamine medication.

Also, make sure you check the ingredients lists on all foods you eat, especially Oriental sauces and pastes, for unexpected shellfish ingredients. Specific ingredients and meals to watch out for if you have a shellfish allergy include:

Bouillabaisse
Caesar salad (dressing normally contains anchovies)
Caponata (a Sicilian relish that can contain anchovies)
Gumbo
Fish sauce
Frito misto

Keeping a Food Diary

To help identify your trigger foods, a *food diary* for a period of time is a great way for you to become aware of what you are eating and the symptoms those foods cause.

For your food diary, you can use a spiral notebook, binder, or folder containing paper—whatever is easiest for you. Write down everything you eat, the approximate size of the serving, and the time. Record both meals and snacks. Next to the food, write down any symptoms you experienced a few minutes to hours after you ate it, and be sure to record the exact time between when you ate the food and when you first experienced symptoms. Be as descriptive as possible. At the end of the week, read through all your foods and symptoms and see if you can make a connection. Make sure you bring your diary to any visits to your family physician or allergist and be ready to report on what you have discovered.

A food diary is effective and easy to put together, but it is only useful if you write down every single food you eat, the time at which you ate it, and the amount. If you occasionally forget to record foods and symptoms, you will never be able to make a true connection between what you eat and how you feel.

Fruits de mer (seafood)
Paella
Kedgeree
Surimi (a processed seafood product, is usually made from white fish, but it can contain some shellfish extract)

SOY ALLERGY

These days, soy is found in an increasing number of foods and food products, from cereals to frozen dinners to canned tuna. While soy allergy usually occurs in children under the age of three, it is becoming more common in teens and adults. Fortunately, soy allergy isn't particularly common overall, affecting only 1 percent of people in the United States; and when it strikes, its symptoms are usually mild.

In rare cases, soy allergies can cause life-threatening anaphylactic reactions, but those usually occur in people who also have a severe peanut allergy and/or asthma.

Symptoms of soy allergy include hives, itching, or eczema; tingling in the mouth; canker sores; swelling of the lips, face, throat, tongue, or other body parts; abdominal pain, diarrhea, nausea, or vomiting; dizziness, lightheadedness, or fainting; and wheezing, trouble breathing, or running nose.

Soy can be hard to avoid because it is used as an ingredient in so many foods and processed food products these days. Some foods that contain hidden soy include baked goods, crackers, infant formulas, sauces, and soups, just to name a few. Because it is so prevalent, you may want to meet with a registered dietitian to discover the best ways to avoid soy in your diet.

As with other allergies, you should check the labels of all foods you eat to make sure they don't contain soy or soy protein. Because labels often use a different name for soy, you should educate yourself on the different soy terms. Here are some of the most common names for soy or soy protein on labels. For maximum safety, carry this list with you at all times:

Akara
Hydrolyzed soy protein
Miso
Soy sauce
Soy grit
Soy nuts
Soy sprouts
Soy protein concentrates
Soy protein isolate
Tamari
Tempeh
Textured vegetable protein
Tofu
Vegetable oil

EGG ALLERGY

Egg allergies can be tough to deal with because eggs show up in far more than the obvious foods, like omelets, soufflé, and egg salad. If you are allergic to eggs, reading labels and asking if foods contain eggs will become part of your daily routine. Egg allergies are similar to other food allergies in that your body overreacts to the egg proteins. Most people with egg allergies are allergic to the proteins in egg whites, but there are also some who cannot tolerate the proteins in the yolk. Egg allergy usually first appears in early childhood and luckily, most kids outgrow it by age five.

If your egg allergy has persisted into your teenage years, you probably know that the symptoms can include hives, eczema, or redness or swelling around your mouth; cramps, diarrhea, nausea, or vomiting; and runny nose, itchy, watery eyes, sneezing, coughing, or asthma. Although it is rare, some people with egg allergy also experience life-threatening anaphylaxis, and in people who are extremely sensitive to eggs, smelling egg fumes or even getting egg on their skin can lead to an anaphylactic reaction.

Because eggs are found in so many foods, if you have an egg allergy, it is a good idea to work with a registered dietitian who can help you develop a safe eating plan. He or she will probably tell you to shop in health food stores, which carry many egg-free products, and to look for vegan foods, which are guaranteed to not contain eggs.

When you eat out at restaurants or at friends' houses, you will have to ask the waitstaff or host if there are any eggs in the foods you are eating; be sure to clearly tell them that you have an allergy and must avoid eggs completely. If your allergy is severe, you should carry an EpiPen or Twinject at all times in case you accidentally come across eggs.

There are studies being conducted at Mt. Sinai School of Medicine that suggest that some people with egg allergies might tolerate very well cooked egg products like food baked with egg in it, but this point is best discussed with an allergist.

For recipes that call for eggs (and let's face it, from brownies to chocolate chip cookies, there are a lot of tasty recipes that do), try the following substitutions for one egg:

- One packet gelatin combined with two tablespoons warm water, mixed right before you are ready to use it
- One teaspoon yeast dissolved in ¼ cup warm water
- One teaspoon baking powder combined with one tablespoon water and one tablespoon vinegar
- One tablespoon pureed fruit, such as bananas or apricots
- Two tablespoons water combined with one tablespoon oil and two teaspoons baking powder

As with other food allergies, you should check the labels of all foods you eat to make sure they don't contain eggs. Because labels often use a different name for eggs and egg products, you should educate yourself on the different terms. Here are some of the most common names for eggs on labels. For maximum safety, carry this list with you at all times:

Albumin
Egg white
Egg yolk
Dried egg
Egg powder
Egg solids
Egg substitutes
Eggnog
Globulin
Livetin
Lysozyme (used in Europe)
Mayonnaise
Meringue
Ovalbumin
Ovomucin
Ovomuciod
Ovovitellin
Simplesse

DIAGNOSING FOOD ALLERGIES

If you haven't yet been diagnosed with a food allergy but you suspect you may have one, see your doctor. He or she will either treat you or refer you to an allergist. The doctor will first ask you questions about how often you experience a reaction, the amount of time that elapses between when you eat the food and when you first have symptoms, and whether or not you have family members with food allergies. Beyond that, doctors use three basic tests to determine whether a person has a food allergy.

Elimination diet. During an *elimination diet,* you will be asked to temporarily eliminate foods to which you may be allergic from your diet. Then your doctor will ask you to slowly reintroduce the foods to see if you experience symptoms. Elimination diets are not used to test for anaphylactic reactions, however, for obvious reasons.

Skin test. During a skin test, liquid extracts of different foods will be placed on your forearm or back and the skin will be pricked lightly to allow the extract to enter your body. If a red, raised spot appears on the area, you are allergic to the food that was placed there. If you take antihistamine medications, you may have to stop taking them two to three days before a skin test so they don't interfere. You may also have to stop taking antidepressants or cold medications, as they too can obstruct the results.

Blood test. Your doctor may also test for food allergy by taking a blood sample and sending it to a lab where it will be mixed with potential allergens and then checked for IgE antibodies. If antibodies are discovered, you have the food allergy.

USING EMERGENCY EPINEPHRINE

Teens with potentially life-threatening food allergies should carry a portable dose of epinephrine with them at all times, as well as directions on how to administer the medication. Portable epinephrine comes in a traditional needle and syringe kit called an *Anakit,* which provides two doses, as well as in an automatic injector system called an EpiPen or Twinject, each of which provide one premeasured dosage. In the event of anaphylactic shock, epinephrine should be injected into the thigh muscle. The medication, which is a synthetic version of the natural hormone adrenaline, works to counteract the anaphylactic reaction; specifically, it acts on the cardiovascular and respiratory systems to reverse throat swelling, constrict blood vessels, stimulate the heart to beat, and relax lung muscles to improve breathing.

No matter which form of epinephrine you use, you should regularly check the expiration date on the medication to make sure it is up-to-date and as potent as possible.

If you have a severe food allergy, in addition to epinephrine your doctor will probably request that you carry a medical alert ID card in your purse or wallet or wear a medical alert bracelet that clearly identifies your allergies.

Beyond the above advice, keep the following in mind:

▸ As soon as you or a friend starts to experience anaphylaxis, call 911. You can start to treat the reaction while you wait for emergency help to arrive, but ultimately, medical assistance is required. Do not attempt to drive yourself or a friend to the hospital.
▸ To administer epinephrine to yourself or a friend, hold the auto injector in the leg for 10 seconds or a slow count of 10.
▸ If symptoms of an anaphylactic attack do not improve, you can give a second dose of epinephrine no sooner than 10–15

minutes after the first one. There is some risk to this amount of epinephrine, however, so this should only be reserved for a severe reaction.

▸ Never try to deal with anaphylaxis by drinking a lot of water in attempt to "flush" the allergen out of your system. This will not work.

▸ If you have a life-threatening food allergy, never attempt to test if a food is safe by touching it with your tongue. While local reactions in the mouth can occur in reaction to a food, they should never be used to determine whether or not a food is safe as they can lead to a full-fledged anaphylactic reaction or falsely lead you to believe that a food does not contain the allergen.

WHAT YOU NEED TO KNOW

▸ Most of the deaths from food allergies occur in teenagers—an indication that teens with food allergies are not being as careful as they should be.

▸ Food allergies differ from other types of allergies in that even a tiny amount of the food—small enough to float through the air—can be fatal.

▸ Although 13 to 18 percent of people in the United States claim to have a food allergy, only 2 percent actually do.

▸ The most common food allergens, which cause 90 percent of food allergies, are milk, eggs, wheat, soy, peanuts and tree nuts, fish, and shellfish.

▸ If one of your parents has a food allergy, your chances of having one yourself are one in three. If both of your parents have food allergies, your odds rise to seven in 10.

▸ Just because you are food allergy–free today doesn't mean that will always be the case. While people are indeed born with a genetic predisposition to allergies, some don't develop symptoms until adulthood.

▸ A food allergy can cause a severe reaction called anaphylaxis, which sets in in as little as five to 15 minutes and leads to itchiness, hives, breathing problems, a sense of impending doom, a drop in blood pressure, a decreased blood flow, especially to the brain, heart, and lungs, and in some cases, death.

▸ If you have a severe food allergy, make sure that you have a Twinject or EpiPen on hand at all times, as well as an over-the-counter antihistamine (antihistamine should be used in addition to an EpiPen or Twinject, not as a replacement).

▸ If you or someone you know has a severe allergic reaction to a food, you should call 911 immediately and administer a dose of epinephrine (EpiPen or Twinject) in the meantime.

▸ If you have a food allergy, whether it is mild, moderate, or severe, the only way to deal with it is to avoid the trigger food(s) and to be on the lookout for symptoms.

▸ Make sure that your family, friends, and acquaintances all know about your allergy, so they can alert you to danger foods and help get you medical attention in the event of an emergency.

▸ Be careful of cross-contamination in your home, which can happen on knives or in the toaster.

▸ Read labels carefully. As of January 2006, food manufactures must state on labels if a food contains one of the eight most common food allergens—milk, eggs, fish, shellfish, peanuts and tree nuts, wheat, and soy.

9

Managing Allergies into the Future

If you are like most teenagers, your sights are set on the future. You often think about what you will do after high school, where you will go to college, and what profession you will choose when you "grow up." If you are a teenager with allergies or asthma, in the midst of all your social and educational planning, you will also have to think about the future of your condition(s), including how their symptoms and management will change as you get older.

As a teen, it is possible that you will outgrow some of the allergies you suffered from as a child; on the other hand, if you were born with a genetic predisposition for allergies, you may also develop *new* allergies as you approach adulthood. No matter whether you are suffering from old allergies or new ones, you must continue to be just as vigilant about controlling your condition as a young adult as you and your parents have been in your teenage years.

This chapter will help you learn what to expect from your allergies as you get older, including how allergies may change in pregnancy and whether or not you will be able to lower your medications in the future. It will also provide useful lifestyle tips on how you can keep your allergies under control into adulthood.

THE DISAPPEARANCE OR DEBUT OF ALLERGIES

Adults usually do not lose their allergies or asthma, but if you are approaching or in the midst of your teenage years, there is still a chance that your springtime sniffling or post-bee-sting swelling may fade away. In addition, if you are currently allergy-free, you can't really count your blessings until you are well into adulthood, as some allergies don't show up until later in life.

The reason some allergies don't show up until adulthood while others disappear is not clearly understood. It seems that people who do not develop allergies until they are older always had a genetic predisposition for them; the genes just didn't "turn on" until later in life. Researchers aren't sure exactly what makes these allergy genes suddenly come alive. Some speculate that the more you are exposed to an allergen—for example, ragweed—the more antibodies to that allergen build up until one day, boom—you have an allergic reaction to ragweed. Once you have that first attack, you will forever have one each time you are exposed to the allergen.

No matter what you are allergic to, as mentioned, there is a chance that it may go away as you approach adulthood or rear its ugly head for the first time on your 18th birthday; and unfortunately, there is no way to predict which will be the case. So the best thing you can do is to be prepared—with the help of the information you have learned in this book—to continue to manage your current allergies diligently as you get older, as well as to be on the lookout for symptoms of allergies that may be yet to develop in the future.

THE FUTURE OF FOOD ALLERGIES

In general, people outgrow the most common food allergies—milk, eggs, wheat, and soy. In fact, 55 percent of kids with these allergies outgrow them by the time they reach age five. Only a small percentage of children with nut and seafood allergies outgrow them, however. The likelihood of outgrowing a food allergy also depends on your symptoms; if you experience eczema or hives after eating a food, you are more likely to outgrow the allergy than if you experience life-threatening anaphylaxis.

It seems the number of times you have encountered a trigger food has an effect on whether you will outgrow your allergy to it as well. Kids with allergies to soy, milk, eggs, and some other allergens can outgrow them if they are careful to avoid these foods in childhood. For example, you will be more likely to outgrow your allergy to eggs if you steer clear of omelets, egg salad, and other egg foods for the first part of your life.

Peanut allergies, which plague an estimated 1 to 2 percent of the population, have long been thought to be lifelong, and in most people, they are, but a recent study shows that a few lucky folks with peanut allergies may outgrow them. The study, conducted at the Division of Allergy and Immunology at the Children's Center at Johns Hopkins University, found that as many as 20 percent of chil-

Keeping an Allergy Diary

No matter what your age, keeping an allergy diary can help you stay abreast of your symptoms so you can figure out what is causing them. Here are some tips on keeping an allergy diary that you can use today and in the future:

➤ Write in your allergy diary every day. This will get you into the habit of using it. If you have no symptoms, record the date and if you want, a quick summary of what you did that day and simply write "no symptoms."

➤ If you have symptoms, write down a detailed account of those symptoms and also record the following:

- Where you were

- What you were doing

- The time of day

- What you wore

- What you ate

- What you touched

➤ If you suspect you have a food allergy, be particularly stringent about recording what you ate. Make sure you write down every food that goes into your mouth, even if it is a snack, and record how you felt after you ate it.

➤ After a few weeks, show the diary to your doctor. He or she will be able to use the information either to make a diagnosis, if you don't already have one, or monitor how your allergy is changing or progressing if you do.

dren outgrow peanut allergies. The researchers recommended that allergists regularly retest patients with peanut allergies to see if their reactions are fading.

The same Johns Hopkins researchers got a similar result when they moved on to tree nuts (almonds, pecans, walnuts, cashews, Brazil nuts, hazelnuts, pine nuts, pistachios, and macadamia nuts). Their follow-up study explored whether tree nut allergies could also be outgrown. They looked at 278 children with tree nut allergies and gave them an oral food challenge—the standard test that proves a child has outgrown a food allergy. Nine percent of the kids passed the challenge, an indication that some children do indeed outgrow tree nut allergies. The study also found that in kids with *both* tree nut and peanut allergies, those who had outgrown their peanut allergies were more likely to also have outgrown their tree nut allergies. Kids with allergies to more than one tree nut were unlikely to outgrow any of their allergies, however.

THE FUTURE OF INSECT ALLERGIES

Kids often outgrow allergies to bee and other insect stings, except when the allergies are severe. A mild reaction to a bee or insect sting involves minor swelling and hives; a severe reaction leads to dizziness, breathing difficulty, and a sudden drop in blood pressure. A study done at Johns Hopkins University showed that children who had serious allergic reactions to bee or other insect stings as kids were likely to have reactions as adults. The good news is that allergy shots can lower your risk of a serious reaction to a bite or sting, even 10 to 20 years after your last shot.

ALLERGIES AND YOUR HORMONES

In your teenage years, you experience a major physiological change in your hormones, and it seems that just as hormones can change your mood, your body hair, and your voice, they can also change your asthma or allergies. For example, up to 40 percent of girls and women with asthma or allergies notice that their symptoms get worse just before menstruation and then improve once their periods are over.

A major consideration if you plan to have children some day is how pregnancy will affect your allergies. If and when you become pregnant, you will probably notice a change in your allergies when you conceive—for the better or for the worse. Just as every pregnant woman has different symptoms in general, every pregnant woman with allergies experiences something unique.

If you have nasal allergies, worsening symptoms won't threaten you or your pregnancy, but they may interfere with your getting a good night's sleep, which is especially important when you are expecting. Therefore, if you notice that your symptoms are getting worse, it is a good idea to stay away from your allergens as much as possible. You will also benefit from staying away from cigarette smoke, perfumes, and other environmental irritants.

If nothing seems to keep your symptoms at bay, there are some allergy medications that you can safely take in pregnancy. Just make sure you discuss any medication you are thinking about taking with your doctor. Here are some specific medications and their safety levels:

Prescription antihistamines: The prescription antihistamine levocetirizine (Xyzal) is classified as category B, but fexofenadine (Allegra) is category C, meaning it should only be used in pregnancy if the benefits outweigh the risks. If you suffer from severe allergies, ask your physician what he or she recommends.

Over-the-counter (OTC) antihistamines: The OTC antihistamines chlorpheniramine (Chlor-Trimeton), diphenhydramine (Benadryl), desloratadine (Clarinex), and cetirizine (Zyrtec) (which is OTC as of January 2008) are classified by the FDA as category B, which means they are considered safe in pregnancy.

OTC decongestants: If you have nasal allergies, you may reach for a decongestant to relieve your stuffy nose. You shouldn't be so fast to do this if you are pregnant, however. The decongestant pseudoephedrine (Sudafed) is classified as category C, so you should avoid taking it during pregnancy, especially in your first trimester. Pseudoephedrine (Sudafed, for example) is now behind the counter because of its abuse to make methamphetamines.

Cromolyn sodium: Originally a source from an Egyptian root, cromolyn sodium (Intal inhalers, Nasal-Crom nose spray, and Crolom eyedrops) is a mast cell stabilizer that is used to prevent allergies. It is classified under the FDA category B. It is one of the safest drugs in the *Physician's Desk Reference.*

Steroids: Nasal steroids are used for environmental allergies, and inhaled steroids are often used to treat asthma. Steroids are classified by the FDA as category C.

Allergy shots: There is no evidence that allergy shots are dangerous in pregnancy, but health-care professionals do not recommend that you get them if you are pregnant. If you are already taking allergy shots and become pregnant, you may be able to continue on your current dose and then stop after you deliver. Ask your physician what he or she recommends.

ASTHMA IN PREGNANCY

Asthma also seems to change during pregnancy. Some women experience worsening asthma symptoms when they are pregnant, and others find that their symptoms improve or stay the same. In some women, asthma can potentially complicate their pregnancies; if it goes uncontrolled, it can lead to serious complications in the mother, including high blood pressure, toxemia, premature delivery, and in rare cases, death. In the fetus, it can lead to risk of stillbirth, premature birth, and low birth weight.

If you have asthma and become pregnant, you can control it with some medications and avoidance of the things that trigger attacks. If you take medication for your asthma, you may be able to continue it when you are pregnant as long as you take it under the supervision of your health-care professional. If possible, you should avoid medications in the first trimester, when the fetus is forming. Inhaled forms are generally preferred because only a small amount of the medication actually gets into the bloodstream. Nursing mothers should take asthma medication at times when they won't be nursing for several hours, however, because most asthma medications enter breast milk.

LIFESTYLE TIPS TO KEEP ALLERGIES UNDER CONTROL

As you approach adulthood, most of the same tactics you used to keep your allergies under control in the past will continue to work for you in the future. Here are some specific ones to keep in mind.

Don't let your sniffles go untreated. Many people try to ignore seasonal allergies, and they spend the entire spring or fall carrying tissues with them wherever they go without ever even talking to a physician. This is a bad idea. If left untreated, seasonal allergies can lead to chronic inflammation of the sinuses (called sinusitis) and asthma. Once you get a proper diagnosis, your physician will prescribe medications to improve your symptoms and overall quality of life, such as antihistamines, topical nasal corticosteroids, cromolyn sodium nasal spray, immunotherapy (allergy shots), or decongestants.

Realize that allergies and asthma are often a dynamic duo. According to the American Academy of Allergies, Asthma & Immunology, up to 78 percent of people who have allergies also have asthma. So if you suffer from allergies, realize that you are also at risk for asthma and discuss your options with your doctor.

If you love your pet, but not your pet allergies, take the necessary steps. Fido and Fluffy may be lovable, but they can wreak havoc if you have allergies. Your beloved pet's dander, skin flakes, saliva, and urine can all create a reaction. Plus, if you have seasonal allergies, your animal may drag the thing you are allergic

Alternative Treatments for Allergies and Asthma

As you get older, you may become more adventurous about trying different treatments for your allergies. This certainly doesn't mean you should use these therapies in lieu of watching out for food allergens, or that you should stop taking your medications if you have a severe allergy. However, if your allergy(s) is mild or moderate, you may want to try some more unconventional therapies. Or, you may want to see what happens when you combine some alternative treatments with your current medications. After all, the following remedies cannot hurt—they can only help. (Note: Never take any vitamin, supplement, or other alternative treatment without checking with your doctor first.)

Vitamin B_6: People with asthma have been found to have lower concentrations of vitamin B_6 (pyridoxine) in their blood, so supplementing with vitamin B_6 (100 milligrams) may help. One study showed that adults with asthma who took 50 milligrams of vitamin B_6 twice a day had improved asthma symptoms and fewer wheezing episodes. Another study showed that kids with asthma who took vitamin B_6 had fewer asthma attacks, less coughing, wheezing, and chest tightness, and a lower requirement of steroid medications.

Magnesium: Magnesium works with calcium to regulate the contraction and relaxation of smooth muscle, so it plays an important role in breathing. People with asthma commonly have low magnesium levels, to—be it mold spores or pollen—into your home, where it will make you sniffle and sneeze. If giving up your pet is simply not an option, do the following to minimize the discomfort he or she is causing:

> ➤ Wash your hands after touching or cuddling with your pet to avoid spreading the dander.
> ➤ Ask someone else to bathe and brush your dog or cat weekly, and have that person brush your pet outdoors several times a week.
> ➤ Keep your pet out of your bedroom.

which makes their condition worse. There have been no conclusive studies on the use of magnesium supplements in people with asthma, but considering the action magnesium has in the body, it just may work.

Zinc: Similar to magnesium, people with asthma have been shown to have lower levels of zinc than those without the condition. Although there have been no definitive studies on the use of zinc supplements in asthmatics, their use appears to be warranted, particularly in preventing asthma symptoms from getting worse.

Omega-3 fatty acids: The omega-3 fatty acids found in fish and nuts appear to do many good things for the body, one being to help decrease inflammation, including inflammation that results from asthma and allergies. Studies have shown that people who eat more fish have a lower risk of asthma. The link isn't quite so clear with omega-3 fatty acid supplements, however. Therefore, in attempt to avoid asthma or decrease your symptoms, it certainly can't hurt to eat fatty fish (like salmon, tuna, or herring) a few times a week.

Massage: Regular massage can help if you have asthma or allergies by reducing anxiety and relaxing your muscles. One study showed that kids with asthma who got daily massage for 30 days experienced an increased peak air flow and higher forced expiratory volume per second.

➤ Store the litter box away from common areas and forced heating and/or air-conditioning vents, and ask someone else to clean it out regularly.

Be on the constant lookout for hidden food allergens. If you have a food allergy, you should be just as diligent about avoiding your trigger foods in your adult years, especially if you are at risk for a life-threatening anaphylactic reaction (a sudden drop in blood pressure that can potentially close air passages and stop the heart). The eight most common food allergens are milk, eggs, peanuts, tree nuts, wheat, soy, fish, and shellfish. Beyond looking for these foods on labels and watching out for them in recipes and at restaurants, beware of the other places they may hide. For example, watch out for deli slicers that are used for both meat and cheese products; milkshakes or smoothies that may contain eggs; ice cream bar toppings that may contain or have been contaminated with nuts; unlabeled ingredients in processed foods; and ethnic dishes that use peanuts or peanut oil.

Escape potential mold traps. If you or someone you love suffers from an allergy to mold, there are some easy things you can do to clean up your environment and therefore decrease your allergies. For one, recognize that mold grows in damp, dark areas of your home and yard; if you have a mold allergy, you should avoid the basement, garden compost piles, and greenhouses. In addition, use a dehumidifier to dry out damp areas; avoid storing clothes, blankets, or frequently used possessions in damp areas; and use a fan or open the bathroom door during steamy showers and baths.

WHAT YOU NEED TO KNOW

➤ As a teen, you may outgrow some of the allergies you suffered from as a child.
➤ If you were born with a genetic predisposition for allergies, you may also develop new allergies as you approach adulthood.
➤ People usually outgrow the most common food allergies—milk, eggs, wheat, and soy. Only a small percentage of children with nut and seafood allergies outgrow them, however.
➤ If you experience eczema or hives after eating a food, you are more likely to outgrow the allergy than if you experience life-threatening anaphylaxis.
➤ A recent study shows that a few lucky folks with peanut allergies may outgrow them. The same researchers got a similar

result when they moved on to tree nuts (almonds, pecans, walnuts, cashews, Brazil nuts, hazelnuts, pine nuts, pistachios, and macadamia nuts).

➤ Kids often outgrow allergies to bee and other insect stings, except when the allergies are severe.

➤ Up to 40 percent of girls and women with asthma or allergies notice that their symptoms get worse just before menstruation and then improve once their periods are over.

➤ If and when you become pregnant, you will probably notice a change in your allergies or asthma when you conceive—for better or worse.

➤ The best thing you can do if you have allergies is to be prepared—with the help of the information you have learned in this book—to continue to manage your current symptoms diligently as you get older, as well as to be on the lookout for symptoms of allergies that may be yet to develop in the future.

10

Helping Friends and Family Cope with Allergies

Many of the people whose lives are touched by allergies have never had a bad reaction to shellfish; they have never spent an entire spring sniffling; and they have never swelled up after a bee sting. In fact, many people who "suffer" from allergies don't have allergies at all; they are friends, family members, camp counselors, and babysitters of children and teenagers who have allergies, and it just as important for these nonallergic folks to know what do to in an allergy emergency as it is for the true sufferers.

If you are a teen who has a friend or family member with allergies, this chapter will help you know what to expect and how to help in the case of an emergency. If you work as a camp counselor or babysitter, this chapter will also help you handle an emergency allergy situation should one arise with one of your clients.

ALLERGIES AND THE FAMILY DYNAMIC

When someone in a family has allergies, it changes the family dynamic, and the more serious the allergies, the more that dynamic changes. If you have a brother or sister with allergies, you probably have felt a range of emotions throughout the years—worry about your sibling, jealousy over the attention that he or she has gotten from your parents, embarrassment because your family is different from others, resentment, and helplessness. If your brother or sister has a food allergy, you have probably been annoyed that your family can't have certain foods at the dinner table. You have probably also felt some of the stress that both your parents and your brother or sister with allergies have dealt with as a result of the condition. All these emotions and experiences are perfectly normal. It is crucial that you do not keep negative emotions bottled up inside—talk to your parents about how you feel on a regular basis.

Although it sometimes may be difficult, one of the best things you can do to help your parents and your sister or brother with allergies is to develop the knowledge necessary to help your sibling, both on a daily basis and in the event of an emergency. After all, it certainly isn't your brother or sister's fault that he or she suffers from allergies; surely, he or she would get rid of the condition if possible. Help your mom or dad get the medication ready for your brother or sister, assist your sibling with reading food labels to make sure foods don't contain allergens, and become educated on the necessary actions so you can assist in the event that your sister or brother suffers an unexpected attack.

Also, be supportive. Activities that some children and teenagers take for granted, such as sports, field trips, and summer camp, are more of a challenge for your brother or sister with allergies, and as a result, he or she probably feels embarrassed and anxious. Encourage your brother or sister to partake in the activities he or she is interested in, but urge him or her to take the necessary precautions. Teenagers are the group of allergy sufferers that take the most risks, so you will do your sibling a huge favor if you remind him or her to have fun, but to be careful.

PREPARING FOR ALLERGY EMERGENCIES

In the midst of an emergency, it can be difficult to think quickly and remember all the things you should do. That is why you cannot be too prepared when an emergency strikes. As someone with an allergic person in your life, be it a friend, sibling, or a child for whom you are responsible, it is a good idea for you to carefully plan what you will do in case an allergy emergency strikes. Here are some actions you can take ahead of time:

Take a health inventory. For a friend, family member, or child you are babysitting or responsible for at camp, ask for a description of the allergies or asthma they have. Make sure you have a list of their allergies to medications and other substances. Also make (or ask for) a list of all the medications the child or teen takes (prescription, over-the-counter, supplements, and herbs), and request insurance coverage information.

Gather all necessary phone numbers. Whether it's for your friend or a family member, make sure you have a list of all relevant phone numbers in case of emergency—parents, doctors, and person to call in an emergency.

Keep first-aid supplies. In case of emergency, it is helpful to have some basic first-aid supplies on hand. These include a thermometer; acetaminophen (Tylenol) or ibuprofen (Motrin or Advil) to reduce fever and/or relieve pain; assorted sizes of bandages; and antibiotic ointment. Additional supplies that may be helpful, depending on the type of allergy attack, include cough syrup; hydrocortisone cream for skin irritations; an elastic bandage; an ice pack; and an over-the-counter antihistamine and decongestant.

Know the most common food allergens. If you work as a baby-sitter or a camp counselor, you should be aware of the most common food allergens. They are peanuts, tree nuts (almonds, cashews, walnuts, pecans, hazelnuts, Brazil nuts), milk, eggs, fish and shellfish, and soybeans. The problem is that these food allergens are not always so obvious—they are often hidden in foods. For example, some hot chocolate is made with peanut butter; some specialty coffees contain tree nuts; tuna is sometimes packed in soy protein; some pasta contains eggs; and skin-care products are occasionally made with crushed shells from nuts or shellfish as an exfoliant.

Be on the lookout for medical alert bracelets. Children or teens who have severe, life-threatening allergies will usually wear medical alert bracelets that clearly state their allergies and, in some cases, what to do in the event of an attack. If you notice that a child you are babysitting or counseling is exhibiting symptoms that may signal anaphylactic shock, check for a medical alert bracelet right away.

Stock up on "safe" snacks. For kids with severe food allergies in your care, keep a stockpile of safe snacks for them to eat. That way you will be able to better control what goes into their mouths and make sure they do not accidentally eat something to which they are allergic.

Learn CPR. You may have to take a cardiopulmonary resuscitation (CPR) certification course if you are babysitting or working as a camp counselor, but even if you're not required, taking a CPR course is a great idea, especially if you have an allergic person in your life. Most local YMCAs and some high schools offer free or low-cost CPR courses.

Don't worry. Worrying about what you will do in the event of an allergy emergency won't help you at all, but preparing will. Instead of stressing out about the potential for an allergy attack in a friend, brother or sister, or child you are babysitting or counseling at camp,

Real-Life Scenario

Chelsea, 17, suffers from a severe peanut allergy. She and her friend Amy, also 17, are inseparable. Because she spends so much time with Amy, Chelsea asked Amy if she would learn how to use her EpiPen injector in case Chelsea accidentally ingested peanuts while the two were together. Of course, Amy agreed. She went over the EpiPen directions several times and examined the device. After about 30 minutes, she was pretty confident that she could administer the emergency epinephrine shot in the event that Chelsea experienced an anaphylactic reaction in her presence.

A few weeks later, Amy was hanging out at the public pool with her younger brother Ed, 12, and her sister Emily, 10. While the three were eating lunch, a yellow jacket stung Emily. Although Emily had experienced swelling after bee stings in the past, this time was much worse. Within a few minutes of the sting, Emily broke out in hives and was having trouble breathing. Amy was scared, but she kept a level head.

"Does anyone have an EpiPen?" she shouted. Luckily, a mother of a nearby boy came running over, EpiPen in hand. Amy quickly administered the dose, using the directions she had memorized at Chelsea's request while the mother called 911. Emily's breathing improved almost immediately, and she recovered from the bee sting completely following a trip to the hospital. She now has her own prescription for an epinephrine kit.

Although Amy learned to use the EpiPen to help her best friend, her knowledge came in handy when she was watching her sister, and she may have saved Emily's life. The moral of the story is that the more people who know how to use an emergency epinephrine device, the better. If you regularly watch younger siblings, or work as a camp counselor or babysitter, the 30 minutes or so that it will take you to learn how to use an EpiPen or Twinject will be very well spent.

channel that energy into learning as much as you can about allergy emergencies and making sure you are trained in all rescue operations possible. Be confident in the fact that if you know what to do, you will handle an emergency with competence.

DEALING WITH AN ALLERGY EMERGENCY

Whether you are the brother or sister of a child or teen with severe allergies, a babysitter, or a camp counselor, there are things you can do to plan for an emergency attack, but you can never be sure exactly how things will play out when one strikes.

Most allergic emergencies are the result of anaphylaxis (also known as anaphylactic shock), a severe allergic reaction that can lead to seizures, cardiac arrhythmia, shock, and in extreme cases, death. Because anaphylaxis is life-threatening, it requires immediate action. Symptoms of anaphylactic shock include difficulty breathing, dizziness, rash, hives, swelling, nausea, vomiting, diarrhea, swollen lips or tongue, wheezing, and low blood pressure. The things that can trigger anaphylaxis include medications, vaccines, food, latex, and insect bites and stings. If your friend, sibling, or a child in your care has encountered a trigger to which they are severely allergic, you will know almost immediately, usually within five to 60 minutes. People with serious allergies can literally be fine one minute and gasping for air the next. So you will have to spring into action quickly.

When an emergency attack occurs in your sibling, if your parents are home, the best thing you can do is to stay calm, quiet, and cooperative, and let your mom and/or dad do what's necessary to help your brother or sister. If that means you have to stay at a friend or neighbor's house while your parents rush your brother or sister to the hospital, so be it.

If you are home alone with your sister or brother, or if the sufferer is a friend or someone under your care, staying calm is also a good first step. If you panic, you will only make the situation worse, both for yourself and the person suffering the attack. Reassure the person having the attack that emergency help is on the way, and tell him or her that you will do everything you can to treat him or her in the meantime. Then have the person sit or lie down in a safe place and remove anything that could hinder his or breathing, such as tight clothing or a foreign object in the mouth, and raise his or her legs. Next, call 911 and alert the hospital of the emergency; that way, an ambulance will be on the way as you administer treatment.

If the person experiencing the attack knows that he or she suffers from anaphylaxis and has an epinephrine kit available (such as an EpiPen or Twinject), you should administer this while emergency help is on the way. An epinephrine kit is a single dose of epinephrine (also known as adrenaline) in a device that resembles a pen. Most reported cases of death from anaphylaxis take place in people who have not received emergency medication, so administering it can literally mean the difference between life and death. Stay with the person until help arrives.

In the event that the emergency attack resulted from an insect bite or sting, first place a tourniquet (a lightly tied band made of cloth or rubber) above the sting site. Remove the tourniquet once every five minutes for a minimum of three minutes, and remove it completely after 30 minutes. Note which type of insect it was, be it a wasp, horsefly, bee, hornet, etc. Knowing the exact circumstances of the attack will help the allergist perform the appropriate tests and, therefore, correctly diagnose the allergy if it hasn't yet been identified.

In some cases of anaphylactic shock, you may have to give your friend, family member, or child in your care a second shot of epinephrine. You will need to give this second shot if the person doesn't improve from the first one, or if he or she starts to experience rebound symptoms before help arrives. Whenever possible, teens with severe allergies with the potential for anaphylaxis should carry two single-shot epinephrine pens in the event of a particularly strong attack.

If the allergic response is less severe, such as hives, and does not include other symptoms, a dose of an oral histamine such as Benadryl may do the trick. You should still seek emergency medical care for the person, however.

Once the person has received emergency treatment, he or she will probably have a follow-up consultation with an allergist, for which information surrounding the attack will be helpful. If the person ate a meal or took a certain medication before he or she suffered the attack, do the following:

- Keep the bottle or box of medication.
- If you know, note how much of the medication the person took.
- Write down all the foods that you know the person ate.
- Keep the labels of any packaged foods the person ate.

Using an EpiPen or Twinject

If you have a friend or family member with a severe allergy who carries an EpiPen or Twinject in case of an emergency, make sure you know how to use the kit before an emergency occurs. Fumbling with the directions and trying to figure out how to administer the medication in the midst of a crisis could lead to an improper dosage. Discuss how to use it with your friend or family member with the allergy, or check out the Web sites of the epinephrine kit to find detailed directions (http://www.twinject.com or http://www.epipen.com). Always check the expiration date on the EpiPen or Twinject before you use it and check its appearance; if it looks discolored or cloudy, it's probably too old. *Adrenaline kits* that have expired lose their potency, and they will not be as effective for your friend or family member.

And remember: Part of being a responsible young adult is readying yourself to handle emergency situations, and this skill is particularly important if you have an allergic person (or persons) in your life. The more you do to prepare for an emergency allergy attack in a friend, family member, or person in your care, the better you will deal with the circumstances when they arise. It cannot be stressed enough that, when it comes to allergies, your actions can literally make the difference between life and death.

CREATING AN EMERGENCY ALLERGY ACTION PLAN

If you work as a babysitter or camp counselor, you want to make sure you are as prepared as possible to handle an allergic emergency should one plague a child in your care. One of the best ways to deal with an emergency is to be ready ahead of time, and an easy way to assure that you are as prepared as possible is to ask parents of the children you are watching to fill out an allergy attack action plan. A sample Emergency Allergy Action Plan may be found in Chapter 5. Here is a letter that you can use as a guideline for the letter you ask parents to fill out, in addition to an action plan:

Sample Letter to Parents from Camp Counselors/Babysitters

Dear Parents or Guardians:

Our camp is/I am prepared to work with you to manage your child's allergy and protect him or her as best as possible. To assure that I/we are as well prepared as possible to deal with an allergy emergency should one occur while your child is in our/my care, I/we ask that you provide the following:

- ► Complete an Emergency Allergy Action Plan (attached) and return it.
- ► Make sure you provide the complete information concerning your child's allergies.
- ► If your child has the potential for anaphylaxis or a serious allergy attack, provide him or her with an EpiPen or Twinject every day he or she is at camp/with me. Make sure that it hasn't expired.

Thank you very much for your cooperation in this important matter. If you have any questions or concerns, please contact _____ at (___)_____.

Child Information

Name: _____

Age: _____

Parents/Guardians: _____

Medications/procedures

Antihistamines _____

Explain dosage and precautions: _____
_____
_____

EpiPen or Twinject_____
_____
_____

Explain administration terms: _____

_____

_____

Other drugs_____

Explain dosage and precautions: _____

_____

_____

AUTHORIZATION AND RELEASE FOR THE ADMINISTRATION OF AN EPIPEN OR TWINJECT

I have requested that an EpiPen be administered in the event of an anaphylaxis emergency. I agree to provide _____ with a written updated medical statement whenever there is a change with respect to medication. I understand that keeping you informed is my responsibility. I also understand that the Emergency Allergy Action Plan will be made available to staff in order to keep everyone informed. Although I know you will work hard to ensure an allergy-free environment, I recognize that you are in no way able to ensure or promise a risk-free or allergen-free experience for my child.

_____
Signature of parent or guardian

_____
Date

WHAT YOU NEED TO KNOW

▸ When someone in a family has allergies, it changes the family dynamic; and the more serious the allergies, the more that dynamic changes.
▸ If you have a sibling with allergies, one of the best things you can do to help your parents and your sister or brother with allergies is to develop the knowledge necessary to help your sibling, both on a daily basis and in the event of an emergency.
▸ Teenagers are the group of allergy sufferers that take the most risks, so you will do your sibling a huge favor if you remind him or her to have fun, but to be careful.

➢ As someone with an allergic person in your life, carefully plan what you will do in case an allergy emergency strikes: know the person's allergies and symptoms; gather all necessary phone numbers; keep first aid supplies on hand; be on the lookout for medical alert bracelets; and learn CPR.

➢ Realize that most allergic emergencies are the result of anaphylaxis (also known as anaphylactic shock), a severe allergic reaction that can lead to seizures, cardiac arrhythmia, shock, and, in extreme cases, death. Symptoms of anaphylactic shock include difficulty breathing, dizziness, rash, hives, swelling, nausea, vomiting, diarrhea, swollen lips or tongue, wheezing, and low blood pressure. The things that can trigger anaphylaxis include medications, vaccines, food, latex, and insect bites and stings.

➢ If your friend or family member is having a serious allergic reaction, have the person sit or lie down in a safe place and remove anything that could hinder his or her breathing, such as tight clothing or a foreign object in the mouth, and raise his or her legs. Next, call 911 and alert the hospital of the emergency; that way, an ambulance will be on the way as you administer treatment.

➢ If the person experiencing the attack knows that he or she suffers from anaphylaxis and has an epinephrine kit available (such as an EpiPen or Twinject), you should administer this while emergency help is on the way.

Paying for Care

Aaron, age 16, has suffered from severe allergic rhinitis
and asthma since he was a small child. From molds to ragweed to
dust, it seems like everything makes him sniffle and sneeze. Luckily, medications and an inhaler have kept Aaron's suffering under
control . . . until recently. Aaron's father's position was eliminated
from his company, rendering him unemployed. As a result, his father
has had to purchase private health insurance, insurance that unfortunately doesn't cover Aaron's expensive medications.

Health-care coverage has become an increasing problem for all
Americans; and for Americans like Aaron and his family who rely on
prescription medications to maintain a good quality of life, the problem is downright scary. Unfortunately, there are far too many teenagers like Aaron whose parents can't afford good health-care coverage
or who make too much money for Medicaid coverage but not enough
to cover medications, doctors' visits, and therapy. Thankfully, there
are some things that Aaron's family and other families like his can
do to get the health-care coverage—and thus, the medical care—that
they need.

Here are some of the options:

HEALTH-CARE COVERAGE

There are many families that do not have adequate health-care coverage these days, for a variety of reasons. Some families are in situations like Aaron's, where the main breadwinner has been laid off.

Others can't afford health-care coverage, or they have jobs that don't offer it, and other families make too much to qualify for state-subsidized health insurance (Medicaid) but too little to pay for private insurance. In addition, some families have health insurance, but they have trouble paying for the high deductibles or co-pays that go along with many health insurance plans these days.

Thankfully, every state in the U.S. has a program specially for infants, children, and teenagers in need of health insurance coverage, called "Insure Kids Now." This program covers doctors' visits, prescription medications, and other services, all for little or no cost. States have different eligibility rules, but most states consider uninsured children ages 18 and younger whose families earn $34,100 or less a year (for a family of four) as eligible. To find out more about "Insure Kids Now" and to see if you and your family are eligible, check out http://www.insurekidsnow.gov or call 1 (877) KIDS-NOW. For more information about immigration status and insurance, go to http://www.ask.hrsa.gov/detail.cfm?id = HRS00291.

Another program that can help you and your family obtain health-care coverage if you are below certain income limits is Medicaid, a state-run public health program that covers a variety of health-care services. Depending on your individual state's rules, Medicaid may require that you make a co-payment (a small part of the fee) for some health-care services; however, all states cover hospital and outpatient care, home health services, and doctor services. To get more information on Medicaid and to find out whether or not you are eligible, you or your parents can go to the Medicaid Web site at http://www.CMS.gov.

COVERAGE FOR MEDICATION COSTS

Medications are the most expensive part of allergy control. Many teenagers with allergies require medication, and some need two, three, or four or more medicines at once. And if you also have asthma, you may need a rescue inhaler as well. Luckily, if controlling your allergy requires that you take expensive prescription medications, you do have options if your parents do not currently have health insurance or a prescription plan.

Many pharmaceutical companies offer free medications to people who cannot afford them. To apply for these free medicines, you will need a note from your doctor stating your need for the medication, as well as a statement declaring that your family has a financial need for the medication or no health insurance or prescription plan to cover it.

To find which companies offer patient assistance, go to the individual companies' Web sites, or you can check out the following Web sites to find out which patients assistance programs offer prescription medications to those in need:

Partnership for Prescription Assistance
(888) 4PPA-NOW (477-2669)
https://www.pparx.org/Intro.php
The Partnership for Prescription Assistance is a combination of doctors, pharmaceutical companies, other health-care providers, community groups, and patient advocacy organizations that help qualify patients without prescription coverage to get the medications they need. The Partnership works with public and private programs and matches them with people who are eligible for free or subsidized medications. Some of the organizations that collaborate on the Partnership for Prescription Assistance include the American Academy of Family Physicians, the American Autoimmune Related Diseases Association, the Lupus Foundation of America, the NAACP, the National Alliance for Hispanic Health, and the National Medical Association.

The Medicine Program
http://www.themedicineprogram.com
The Medicine Program offers a free discount drug program to large groups and corporations. The program is available to anyone who wants to lower the cost of his or her prescription medications. The free prescription card, which is accepted at more than 35,000 participating pharmacies, can save you up to 60 percent off your prescription medications.

NeedyMeds
http://www.needymeds.com
NeedyMeds is a database of patient assistance programs that helps people obtain health supplies, medication, and equipment. The site, which was created by Libby Overly, M.Ed., MSW, a former social worker from Alabama, and Richard J. Sagall, M.D., helps patients in need to obtain free drugs, discount drugs, and other medical supplies. A free site, NeedyMeds has been helping patients find subsidized medications since 1997, and the site is constantly being updated with new information. If you would prefer a hard copy, you can also get The NeedyMeds Manual, *which contains all the valuable information from the web site.*

RxAssist

http://www.rxassist.org

A comprehensive database of patient assistance programs run by pharmaceutical companies, RxAssist helps people who cannot afford medications to obtain free medicines. In addition, the site offers news, practical tools, and articles to help health-care professionals and patients find necessary information.

Free Medicine Foundation

http://www.freemedicinefoundation.com

The volunteer-run Free Medicine Foundation helps families like Aaron's to eliminate or significantly lower their prescription medication costs. In fact, the Free Medicine Foundation helps the average member save $890 per year on each medication that he or she takes. The organization works by helping people get free medicine directly from pharmaceutical sponsors. If your family has no prescription coverage, a low income, or maxed-out prescription benefits, you are eligible to apply. Individuals with family incomes from the poverty level to $38,000, and families with annual incomes as high as $80,000 can get free medications. However, keep in mind that each sponsored drug has its own eligibility criteria.

MEDICATIONS FROM CANADA

As medications and health-care coverage in general become more expensive and harder to get, there is more and more buzz about people buying their drugs from Canada. As much as the U.S. government may dislike this practice—in part because there is no way to regulate these drugs and assure that they are safe—many consumer advocates say it's an economical way to obtain expensive medications. Should you and your parents decide to get your medications from Canada, make sure you are getting them from a reputable Web site. As the practice of buying medications from Canada becomes more popular, several states have developed programs to help their residents obtain medications from Canada, and these sites have been deemed safe.

One such site is http://www.i-saverx.net, an easy-to-use mail-order pharmacy program that can save you money on medications if you live in the states of Kansas, Illinois, Missouri, Vermont, or Wisconsin. The governors of these states developed this program to help provide their residents with lower-cost brand prescription drugs from Canada, Ireland, and the United Kingdom.

In addition, Minnesota, North Dakota, and New Hampshire have all set up programs to help residents obtain lower-priced drugs from foreign countries. Here are their specific programs:

Minnesota

To help residents find discounted drugs from Canada and the United Kingdom, the governor of Minnesota set up a Web site called Minnesota RXConnect online. For more information, check out the site at http://www.state.mn.us/portal/mn/jsp/home.do?agency = Rx.

North Dakota

To help North Dakota residents obtain lower-priced drugs from Canada, the following Web site provides links to Web sites that import discounted medications from abroad. For more information, check out the site at http://www.governor.state.nd.us/prescription-drugs.html.

New Hampshire

New Hampshire helps its residents find discounted medications with a number of helpful sites, including a link to CanadaDrugs.com. For more information, check out http://www.egov.nh.gov/medicine%2Dcabinet.

WHAT YOU NEED TO KNOW

‣ If your family doesn't have an adequate health insurance and/ or prescription plan, you have options.

‣ Every state has a program that offers health insurance to children and teenagers in need, and there are a number of programs that offer free or discounted prescription medications.

‣ If your family is below a certain income level, you may be eligible for Medicaid, a state program that offers health-care coverage to those in need.

‣ Some states provide Web sites for residents that explain how to obtain lower-priced medications abroad.

‣ If you are having a serious allergy attack, you will be examined and treated at an emergency room, even if you don't have insurance or cannot pay for the services.

APPENDIX

Associations and Resources

Allergy & Asthma Network/Mothers of Asthmatics (AANMA)
2751 Prosperity Avenue, Suite 150
Fairfax, VA 22031
(800) 878-4403
(703) 573-7794 (fax)
http://www.aanma.org

The Allergy Institute
7375 N. Fresno Street
Fresno, CA 93720
(559) 447-1700
http://www.allergyinstitute.com

The American Academy of Allergy, Asthma & Immunology
555 East Wells Street, Suite 1100
Milwaukee, WI 53202-3823
(414) 272-6071
http://www.aaaai.org

American Latex Allergy Association
3791 Sherman Road
Slinger, WI 53086
(888) 972-5378
(262) 677-0324 (fax)
alert@latexallergyresources.org
http://www.latexallergyresources.org

American Partnership for Eosinophilic Disorders
3419 Whispering Way Drive
Richmond, TX 77469
(713) 498-8216
apfed@sbcglobal.net
http://www.apfed.org

Asthma & Allergy Foundation of America
122 20th Street NW, Suite 402
Washington, DC 20036
(800) 7-ASTHMA [727-8462]
info@aafa.org
http://www.aafa.org

Centers for Disease Control and Prevention:
   Asthma and Allergies
http://www.cdc.gov/health/asthma.htm

Food Allergy & Anaphylaxis Network
11781 Lee Jackson Highway, Suite 160
Fairfax, VA 22033-3309
(800) 929-4040
http://www.foodallergy.org

Food Allergy Initiative
1414 Avenue of the Americas, Suite 1804
New York, NY 10019
(212) 207-1974
(917) 338-5130 (fax)
http://www.foodallergyinitiative.org

The Food Allergy Project
(212) 681-1380
FoodAllergyInfo@FoodAllergyProject.org
http://www.foodallergyproject.org

Immune Deficiency Foundation
25 West Chesapeake Avenue, Suite 206
Towson, MD 21204
(800) 296-4433
(410) 321-9165 (fax)
http://www.primaryimmune.org

Kids with Food Allergies
73 Old Dublin Pike, Suite 10, #163
Doylestown, PA 18901
(215) 230-5394
(215) 340-7674 (fax)
http://www.kidswithfoodallergies.org

National Allergy Bureau
Manager, National Allergy Bureau
AAAAI Executive Office
555 E. Wells Street, 11th Floor
Milwaukee, WI 53202-3823
(414) 272-6071
nab@aaaai.org
http://www.aaaai.org/nab
Compiles pollen and mold counts as reported by certified stations
across the country and announces them each week on the NAB
page of the AAAAI's Web site.

SchoolAsthmaAllergy.com
http://www.schoolasthma.com

SUPPLIERS OF ALLERGY-FREE FOOD PRODUCTS
The Gluten-Free Pantry
(800) 291-8386
http://www.glutenfree.com

Miss Roben's
Allergy Grocer
91 Western Maryland Parkway, Unit #7
Hagerstown, MD
(800) 891-0083
http://www.missroben.com

GLOSSARY

acrivastine and pseudoephedrine   A prescription decongestant/ antihistamine combination. Brand name is Semprex-D.

adrenaline   Also called epinephrine. A fast-acting medicine that helps offset an anaphylactic reaction.

adrenaline kit   An emergency kit that contains adrenaline and other allergy medication for use in a sudden, unexpected exposure to an allergen that causes life-threatening symptoms.

Advair   A bronchodilator (salmeterol)/corticosteroid combination that is available in a disk-shaped metered dose contraption called a "Diskus."

Afrin   An over-the-counter (OTC) decongestant nasal spray.

albuterol   A short-acting, immediate-relief bronchodilator. Brand names are Proventil HFA and ProAir HFA.

allergen   A substance that causes an allergy attack.

allergist   A physician trained in the prevention, diagnosis, and treatment of problems involving the immune system, including allergies.

allergy   An abnormal immune system response to a substance (allergen) that would otherwise be harmless.

allergy shots   Shots that give you a small dose of the substance to which you are allergic. Common allergies treated with allergy shots include those to weeds, mold, pollen, grasses, dust mites, household pets, and trees.

Anakit   Portable epinephrine in a traditional needle and syringe kit.

anaphylactic shock   A severe and sometimes fatal reaction in a susceptible person after exposure to a specific allergen (e.g., food, pollen, proteins in latex gloves, or penicillin). Also called anaphylaxis.

anaphylactoid reaction   A reaction that is just as serious as anaphylaxis but does not involve IgE antibodies. Allergens that can cause anaphylactoid reactions include fish, latex, and some medications, like penicillin.

anaphylaxis   See *anaphylactic shock.*

antibodies Proteins the immune system produces in response to a foreign substance (antigen).

antihistamine A drug given to reduce or reverse an allergic reaction.

antihistamine-decongestant combinations: Medications that target allergies by blocking histamine and also treating the runny nose, nasal congestion, and sneezing that accompany some allergies (usually hay fever).

asthma A narrowing of airways in the lungs that leads to coughing, wheezing, and shortness of breath.

asthma action plan A plan developed by your physician to guide you in the ongoing treatment of your asthma.

azelastine A new antihistamine nasal spray used to treat seasonal allergies. Brand name is Astelin.

Beconase A corticosteroid nasal spray.

Benadryl An OTC antihistamine.

bronchodilators Medications that keep your airways open by relaxing the bronchial muscles.

cetirizine A prescription-strength antihistamine. Brand name is Zyrtec.

cetirizine HCL A prescription-strength antihistamine/decongestant combination. Brand name is Zyrtec-D.

chest X-ray A test used to rule out diseases such as pneumonia or a sinus disease that may be causing allergy symptoms.

Chlor-Trimeton An OTC antihistamine.

Claritin An OTC antihistamine.

complete blood count (CBC) A test to check the number of red blood cells, white blood cells, and platelets in a sample of blood.

conjunctivitis Also known as pink eye. Inflammation of the membrane that lines the eyelids and covers the surface of the eyeball

corticosteroids Drugs that help reduce the inflammation, stuffiness, runny nose, sneezing, and itching due to both seasonal and year-round allergies. They can also reduce swelling and inflammation from other types of allergic reactions. Corticosteroids come in a number of forms, depending on the type of allergy they are being used to treat, including pills, nasal sprays, inhalers, and eyedrops.

cromolyn sodium A type of medicine called a mast cell stabilizer. When mast cells in the nose encounter an allergen, they release histamine, which unleashes sniffling, sneezing, and other allergy symptoms. Cromolyn sodium and other mast cell stabilizers prevent the mast cells from releasing histamine in the first place, so you never experience the annoying symptoms.

cross-contamination   This occurs when a "safe" food touches a food allergen, such as on a knife or in the toaster, and then produces a resulting allergic reaction.

CT (CAT) scan   A test that creates a detailed image of your sinuses to rule out a chronic sinus problem.

cytokine   A chemical messenger produced by white blood cells that helps carry out immune functions.

dander   Minute scales of hair, feathers, or skin.

decongestant   A drug used to relieve congestion and swelling in the nose and sinuses.

dehumidifier   A device that helps to remove excess moisture from the air.

dermatologist   A doctor specially trained to diagnose and treat skin problems.

desloratadine   An OTC antihistamine. Brand name is Clarinex.

dexamethasone   A prescription eyedrop corticosteroid. Brand name is Tobradex.

Dimetane   An OTC antihistamine. Includes a combination of brompheniramine maleate, phenylpropanolamine hydrochloride, and codeine phosphate.

double-blind food challenge   A test for food allergies. During this test, which is only done if your reactions are not severe, you will swallow a series of capsules containing various potential triggers one at a time, and neither you nor your doctor will know which capsule contains the substance you are allergic to. After you swallow each capsule, the doctor will watch to see if you experience a reaction.

dust   A mixture of lots of different things found in your home— fibers from carpeting and drapes, food remnants, pet hair, pet dander, debris from furniture, and outside dust from traffic or nearby construction sites.

dust mites   Tiny critters that cause allergies. Dust mites can be found anywhere there is dust—in bedding, mattresses, upholstered furniture, and carpeting.

eczema   A skin condition that causes areas of the skin to become red, itchy, and scaly.

elimination diet   A diet during which you temporarily eliminate foods to which you may be allergic. Foods are then slowly reintroduced to see if you experience symptoms.

elimination tests   Tests during which your physician asks you to avoid certain substances or foods to see if you improve.

epinephrine   Also called adrenaline. A fast-acting medicine that helps offset an anaphylactic reaction.

EpiPen   An epinephrine auto-injector. In the event of an attack, you inject the medication into the front of your thigh, and the injection immediately relaxes your narrowed airways and raises your blood pressure by constricting your small blood vessels.

fexofenadine   A prescription-strength antihistamine. Brand name is Allegra.

fexofenadine HCl   A prescription-strength antihistamine decongestant combination. Brand name is Allegra-D.

Flonase   A corticosteroid nasal spray.

Flovent   An inhaled corticosteroid used to treat asthma.

fluticasone   A prescription nasal spray used to treat allergies. Brand name Flonase.

food diary   A diary in which you write down every single food you eat, the time at which you ate it, the amount, and any symptoms you experience.

hay fever   A seasonal type of allergic rhinitis caused by pollen. Hay fever is characterized by itching and tearing of the eyes, swelling of the nasal mucosa, sneezing, and often, asthma.

HEPA filter   Stands for high efficiency particulate arresting (HEPA) filter. A HEPA filter will help remove allergens from the air in your bedroom, including dust, pet dander, or mold spores.

histamine   A substance released by the mast cells during an allergic reaction. It causes itching, sneezing, increased mucous production, and nasal congestion,

hives   Itchy, swollen, red bumps or patches on the skin that appear suddenly as a result of the body's reaction to certain allergens.

Hymenoptera   Insects with biting jaws and usually four wings. They include bees and yellow jackets.

IgE antibodies   Special proteins the body makes in response to substances it thinks are harmful. IgE antibodies are produced when one is exposed during an allergic reaction, and they lead to inflammation.

immune system   The complicated group of organs and cells that defends the body against foreign substances, such as bacteria or allergens, by producing antibodies.

immune system tests   Tests that measure the functioning of your immune system. The catchall test of the immune system is the complete blood count, which measures your white blood cell count, your platelets (substances in your blood that help it clot), and your hematocrit (the concentration of your blood). This test can be broken down further to look at levels of specific white blood cells, including lymphocytes, neutrophils, eosinophils, and basophils. Another common test involves measuring immunoglobulin levels (IgG, IgA, IgM, and IgE).

immunotherapy   Allergy shots. Similar to a vaccine, an allergy shot gives you a small dose of the substance to which you are allergic. Common allergies treated with immunotherapy include those to weeds, mold, pollen, grasses, dust mites, household pets, and trees.

indoor air pollution   Pollution inside your home. Common causes of indoor air pollution include cigarette smoke, natural gas, cosmetics, glue, ammonia, perfumes, gasoline, motor oil, nail polish, and detergents.

inflammatory   A localized protective reaction of tissues to irritation, infection, or injury characterized by redness, swelling, and pain.

ketotifen fumarate   A prescription antihistamine decongestant combination. Brand name is Zaditor.

lactose   A sugar present in milk.

latex   An emulsion of rubber or plastic globules in water used in paints, adhesives, rubber gloves, and various synthetic rubber products.

leukotrienes   Inflammatory substances that are released by mast cells during an allergic response or asthma attack.

loratadine/pseudoephedrine sulfate   A prescription decongestant. The brand name is Claritin-D.

loteprednol   A prescription eyedrop corticosteroid. Brand name is Alrex.

mast cell   A type of white blood cell. The contents of the mast cells, along with those of basophils, are responsible for the symptoms of allergy.

Medic Alert bracelet or necklace   Devices that are engraved with your medical condition, membership number, and a 24-hour emergency response number.

mold   A microscopic fungi that lives off of decaying plant life.

mometasone   A prescription nasal spray used to treat allergies. Brand name is Nasonex.

montelukast   A medication that helps to ease the symptoms of asthma as well as both indoor and outdoor allergies. Brand name is Singulair.

naphazoline hydrochloride   A prescription antihistamine/decongestant combination. Brand names include Naphcon and Vasocon.

nasal sprays   Medicines used to prevent and treat nasal allergy symptoms. Nasal sprays are available by prescription or over-the-counter in decongestant, corticosteroid, or salt-water solution forms.

Nasocort   A corticosteroid nasal spray.

Nasonex   A corticosteroid nasal spray.

Neo-Synephrine   An OTC decongestant nasal spray.

oral challenge   A test during which you get small doses of various substances and are then monitored for allergy symptoms such as hives, wheezing, or a drop in blood pressure.

otolaryngologist   A physician who specializes in diseases of the ears, nose, throat, head, and neck. Also called an ear, nose, and throat (ENT) physician.

outdoor air pollution   Pollution that occurs outdoors. The biggest source of outdoor air pollution is smog, the heavy, gray cloud of air pollution that hangs over most major cities. This is not only an eyesore on otherwise pretty skylines but it can trigger allergies. In sensitive people, smog can cause breathing problems, eye irritation, tiredness, and other symptoms.

over-the-counter (OTC)   Products sold at local drugstores and other stores without a prescription.

patch test   A test to discover which allergen is responsible for contact dermatitis in a patient. Low concentrations of different allergens are applied under a patch on the back. A positive test will show a skin reaction.

peak flow measurement   Measurement of the maximum rate of airflow. To perform the test, you blow into a handheld device that gives you a reading called a peak flow rate, usually given in liters per minute.

peak flow meter   A portable handheld device that measures your ability to push air out of your lungs.

peanut allergy   A type of food allergy, distinct from tree nut allergies, that causes an overreaction of the immune system. Peanut allergies can cause life-threatening anaphylactic reactions.

pet allergy   A hypersensitivity to pets that causes an overreaction of the immune system. Symptoms of pet allergies include sneezing, itchy, watery eyes, and congestion. The most common household pets are dogs, cats, birds, hamsters, rabbits, mice, gerbils, rats, and guinea pigs, all of which can cause allergies.

pH probe test   A test done to rule out gastroesophageal reflux disorder (GERD), a condition in which your stomach acid travels upward into your esophagus. A pH probe test measures the stomach acid in your esophagus for 24 hours.

pimecrolimus   A topical medication used to treat skin eczema. Brand name is Elidel.

pollen Tiny, egg-shaped male cells of flowering plants. Although they are small—no wider than the average human hair—they can pack a big wallop when it comes to allergies.

prednisone An oral prescription corticosteroid. Brand names are Prednisone Intensol, Sterapred, and Sterapred DS.

pseudoephedrine An ingredient in decongestants. The most popular OTC decongestant is Sudafed. However, most pharmacies keep all medications with pseudoephedrine behind the counter these days.

Pulmicort An inhaled corticosteroid used to treat asthma.

pulmonary function test A test for asthma. To do the test, you will blow into a machine that measures your breathing before and after you use an inhaler. If your breathing improves after using the inhaler, you probably indeed have asthma.

pulmonologist A physician who specializes in the treatment of lung disease.

radioallergosorbent test (RAST) The most common blood test used for allergies.

ragweed Any of a variety of North American weedy herbs that produce pollen and are highly allergenic.

respiratory system The organs that are involved in breathing, including the nose, throat, larynx, trachea, bronchi, and lungs.

rheumatologist A physician who studies, diagnoses, and treats arthritis and other diseases of the joints, muscles, and bones.

rhinitis Inflammation of the mucous membrane inside the nose.

Rhinocort A corticosteroid nasal spray.

skin test A test during which extracts of different foods are placed on your forearm or back and the skin is pricked lightly to allow the extract to enter your body; if a red, raised spot appears on the area, you are allergic to the food that was placed there.

spirometry A pulmonary function test.

steroid A type of drug used to relieve swelling and inflammation.

Sudafed An OTC decongestant.

Symbicort An inhaled corticosteroid/bronchodilator combination used to treat asthma.

tacrolimus A topical medication used to treat skin eczema. Brand name is Protopic.

Tavist An OTC antihistamine.

TNX-901 A drug currently being studied that may prevent peanut allergies by blocking IgE, the substance that starts the allergic reaction chain.

triamcinolone A prescription nasal spray used to treat allergies. Brand names are Nasacort AQ, Azmacort.

Twinject An epinephrine auto-injector. In the event of an attack, you inject the medication into the front of your thigh, and the injection immediately relaxes your narrowed airways and raises your blood pressure by constricting your small blood vessels.

wheezing Continuous, coarse, whistling sounds produced in the respiratory airways during breathing when the airways are constricted.

READ MORE ABOUT IT

Berger, William E., M.D. *Allergies and Asthma for Dummies.* Foster City, Calif.: IDG Books Worldwide, 2000.

Bock, Steven J., M.D., and Kenneth Bock, M.D. *Natural Relief for Your Child's Asthma: A Guide to Controlling Symptoms & Reducing Your Child's Dependence on Drugs.* New York: HarperPerennial, 1999.

Dozor, Allen, and Kate Kelly. *The Asthma and Allergy Action Plan for Kids: A Complete Program to Help Your Child Live a Full and Active Life.* New York: Fireside, 2004.

Ehrlich, Paul, M.D., and Larry Chiaramonte, M.D. *What Your Doctor May Not Tell You About Children's Allergies and Asthma: Simple Steps to Help Stop Attacks and Improve Your Child's Health.* New York: Warner Books, 2003.

Farber, Harold, and Michael Boyette. *Control Your Child's Asthma: A Breakthrough Program for the Treatment and Management of Childhood Asthma.* New York: Holt Paperbacks, 2001.

The Food Allergy & Anaphylaxis Network. *Stories From the Heart: A Collection of Essays from Teens with Food Allergies.* Fairfax, Va.: Food Allergy & Anaphylaxis Network, 2002.

The Food Allergy & Anaphylaxis Network. *Stories from Parental Hearts: Essays by Parents of Children with Food Allergies.* Fairfax, Va.: Food Allergy & Anaphylaxis Network, 2004.

Jaggi, O. P. *Positive Options for Children with Asthma: Everything Parents Need to Know.* Alameda, Calif.: Hunter House, 2005.

May, Jeffrey C. *My House Is Killing Me!: The Home Guide for Families with Allergies and Asthma.* Baltimore: The Johns Hopkins University Press, 2001.

Pescatore, Fred. *The Allergy and Asthma Cure: A Complete Eight-Step Nutritional Program.* Hoboken, N.J.: Wiley, 2003.

Plaut, Thomas F., M.D., with Teresa Jones, M.A. *Dr. Tom Plaut's Asthma Guide for People of All Ages.* Amherst, Mass.: Pedipress, 1999.

Rachelefsky, Gary, and Patricia Garrison. *Free Your Child from Asthma.* New York: McGraw Hill, 2005.

Welch, Michael J., M.D. *American Academy of Pediatrics Guide to Your Child's Allergies and Asthma: Breathing Easy and Bringing Up Healthy, Active Children.* New York: Villard, 2000.

Wray, Betty B., M.D. *Taking Charge of Asthma: A Lifetime Strategy.* New York: John Wiley & Sons, 1998.

INDEX